A THERAPIST'S MANUAL FOR COGNITIVE BEHAVIOR THERAPY IN GROUPS

A THERAPIST'S MANUAL FOR COGNITIVE BEHAVIOR THERAPY IN GROUPS

Lawrence I. Sank and Carolyn S. Shaffer

Center for Cognitive Therapy
Bethesda, Maryland

The George Washington University Medical Center
Washington, D.C.

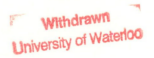
PLENUM PRESS • NEW YORK AND LONDON

Library of Congress Cataloging in Publication Data

Sank, Lawrence, I., date–
   A therapist's manual for cognitive behavior therapy in groups.

   Bibliography: p.
   Includes index.
   1. Behavior therapy—Handbooks, manuals, etc. 2. Cognitive therapy—Handbooks, manuals, etc. 3. Group psychotherapy—Handbooks, manuals, etc. I. Shaffer, Carolyn S., 1946–   . II. Title. [DNLM: 1. Behavior therapy—Methods. 2. Cognition. 3. Psychotherapy, Group—Methods. WM 430 S277t]
RC489.B4S175 1983   616.89'152   83-13652
ISBN 0-306-41229-2

© 1984 Plenum Press, New York
A Division of Plenum Publishing Corporation
233 Spring Street, New York, N.Y. 10013

Printed in the United States of America

We dedicate this volume to
those who have so patiently supported us
throughout the development of this program and
the writing of this book:
Jim, Linda, Jessica, Benjamin, and David.

FOREWORD

One of the great advantages of rational-emotive therapy (RET) and cognitive behavior therapy (CBT) is that they frequently employ psychoeducational methods—including bibliotherapy, workshops, lectures, courses, recordings, and films. I created RET at the beginning of 1955 after I had abandoned the practice of psychoanalysis because I found it to be highly inefficient and philosophically superficial. Being almost addicted to one-to-one therapy as a result of my analytic training and experience, I at first did RET only with individual clients and found this pioneering form of CBT considerably more effective than the other therapies with which I had experimented.

By 1957, however, I realized that RET could be taught to large numbers of persons through self-help books and articles and that RET-oriented writings could not only prove valuable to the general public but that they could also be successfully employed to hasten and intensify the therapy of my individual clients. I therefore wrote a number of RET self-help books—especially *How to Live with a Neurotic* (1957), *Sex without Guilt* (1958), *A New Guide to Rational Living* (with Robert A. Harper; original edition, 1961), and *A Guide to Successful Marriage* (with Robert A. Harper, 1961). The effectiveness of these books has surpassed my wildest expectations—since they have sold millions of copies (notably in the paperback editions published by Wilshire Book Company, North Hollywood, California), have been recommended to clients by hundreds of therapists, have been translated into more than twenty foreign languages, have brought to my mailbox and to my face thousands of enthusiastic testimonials, and have encouraged the publication of many other CBT-oriented self-help books, such as Robert Alberti and Michael Emmons's *Your Perfect Right*, Wayne Dyer's *Your Erroneous Zones*, and David Burns's *Feeling Good*.

Spurred on by the psychoeducational success of *How to Live with a Neurotic* and *A New Guide to Rational Living*, I began in 1959 to apply RET to group therapy and to large-scale workshops. Again, it seemed to work significantly better than conventional therapies do when used in group form. I have now seen about 2,500 regular group-therapy clients during the last 24 years (since I lead 6 groups every week, each of which has a maximum of 13 clients) and have given over a thousand RET workshops to well over one hundred thousand people during this same period. Following my lead, the Institute for Rational-Emotive Therapy in New York, which I direct, and its allied branches and groups throughout the world now give hundreds of other RET workshops every year, and many other CBT therapists and centers (such as the Center for Cognitive Therapy in Philadelphia and in Bethesda, Maryland) give innumerable other CBT-oriented talks, workshops, and other public presentations.

All of which indicates—what? Presumably, that RET and CBT are not merely effective therapies on a one-to-one basis, but that they also have important group and psychoeducational applications. That is why this book by Lawrence I. Sank and Carolyn S. Shaffer, *A Therapist's Manual for Cognitive Behavior Therapy in Groups*, is such a valuable volume. It takes four of the major aspects of CBT—relaxation training, cognitive restructuring, assertion training, and problem solving—and it shows in great detail how these methods can be used in a brief group-therapy format. It tells the therapist who would employ these modes of CBT exactly how to do so over a period of 15 weekly sessions. And it provides suitable handouts, bibliotherapy suggestions, and other materials that therapists of CBT groups can use to help themselves and their group members. It is remarkably complete in these aspects, and it is written in such a clear and simple manner, with a minimum of technical jargon, that virtually all therapists or counselors who want to use group CBT techniques can distinctly follow its procedures and add to their knowledge and their skills.

Is *A Therapist's Manual for Cognitive Behavior Therapy in Groups* thoroughly comprehensive and flawless? Of course not. It only briefly mentions, for example, several important cognitive methods—such as modeling, philosophical analysis, and the use of humor. It is skimpy in its employment of emotive-evocative techniques, such as rational-emotive imagery, forceful self-statements, and RET's famous shame-attacking exercises. But since cognitive behavior therapy now includes literally hundreds of possible methods, and since no book is likely to be truly comprehensive in explaining all of them, Drs. Sank and Shaffer cannot legitimately be faulted for not being all things to all readers.

What the book does contain is distinctly good. It is hard-headed, practical, and right down to earth. It presents a CBT program that can be easily understood and utilized. It can be selectively used and discriminatingly modified by those therapists who want to experiment with and add to or subtract from it. Like RET and CBT themselves, it presents no dogmas or unfalsifiable assumptions. Sank and Shaffer's book is a welcome addition to the CBT literature. I predict good results for the therapists and clients who work at using it.

ALBERT ELLIS, PH.D.
Executive Director
Institute for Rational-Emotive Therapy
45 East 65th Street
New York, New York 10021

CONTENTS

FOREWORD vii
Albert Ellis

INTRODUCTION   1

Chapter 1
COPING SKILLS TRAINING AND COGNITIVE BEHAVIOR
THERAPY   9
Thomas L. McKain

Chapter 2
THE SCREENING PROCEDURE 25

Chapter 3
THE RELAXATION MODULE 41

    Session 1 41
    Session 2 49

Chapter 4
THE COGNITIVE RESTRUCTURING MODULE 63

    Session 3 63

Chapter 5
ENHANCING COGNITIVE RESTRUCTURING SKILLS 77

    Session 4 77
    Session 5 91
    Session 6 99

Chapter 6
INDIVIDUAL SESSION / MIDWAY EVALUATION 107

    Session 7 107

Chapter 7
THE ASSERTION-TRAINING MODULE 113

    Session 8 113
    Session 9 125
    Session 10 133
    Session 11 141

Chapter 8
THE PROBLEM-SOLVING MODULE 149

    Session 12 149
    Session 13 157

Chapter 9
CLOSING SESSIONS 165

    Session 14 167
    Session 15 171

Chapter 10
BOOSTER SESSIONS 177

REFERENCES 181

APPENDIXES 187

    1. Pretreatment Questionnaire (PTQ) 187
    2. Pregroup Screening Description of the Coping Skills
       Group 199
    3. List of Symptoms Common to Patients Referred to the
       Coping Skills Group 201
    4. Potential Goals for Each Module 203

 5. Coping Skills Group Screening Form—Individual Goal
    Sheet   205
 6. Coping Skills Group Attendance/Performance Record
    and Contract   207
 7. Example of Completed Coping Skills Group Screening
    Form—Individual Goal Sheet   209
 8. Relaxation Practice Log   211
 9. List of Required and Suggested Readings   213
10. Personal Reminder Form   215
11. Example of Completed Personal Reminder Form   217
12. Relaxation Sequence   219
13. Cognitive Distortions   221
14. Dispute Handles   223
15. Homework Sheet for Cognitive Restructuring   225
16. Advanced Homework Sheet for Cognitive Restructuring   227
17. Therapist's Example   229
18. Basic Irrational Ideas   231
19. Homework Sheet for Cognitive Restructuring   233
20. CBT Homework Sheet: Example Originally Prepared for
    Nondisclosure to Group   235
21. CBT Homework Sheet: Example Done at Home That
    Prompted Self-Disclosure in the Group   239
22. Components of Assertive Behavior   241
23. Scripted Assertive Scenes   243
24. Vignettes for Assertiveness Training   245
25. Assertive Behavior Log   249
26. Problem-Solving Homework Sheet   251
27. Completed Problem-Solving Homework Sheet   253
28. Example of Completed Goal Sheet for Final Interview   255
29. Worksheet for Remaining Problems   257
30. Individual Goal Sheet for Final Interview   259
31. Log of Problem Situations and Skills Employed   261

INDEX   263

INTRODUCTION

This manual is designed to provide the experienced mental health practitioner with an easy-to-read, easily followed guide to the treatment of anxiety and depression in a brief group therapy format. The techniques of relaxation, assertiveness, cognitive restructuring, and problem solving compose what we have come to call the Coping Skills Program. This program was developed over a span of seven years at the George Washington University Health Plan, a health maintenance organization (HMO) functioning within the George Washington University Medical Center in Washington, D.C. Our goal was to develop a brief, time-limited, cost-effective means of teaching important self-help skills to moderately anxious or depressed patients. These patients were either self-referred or referred by primary care medical providers.

THE PRACTITIONER

This program is designed for the professional with clinical experience or the graduate-level trainee working under the guidance of an experienced supervisor. Experience with behavior or cognitive/behavior therapy would prove helpful in working with this manual, as would group therapy experience. However, we have not, in our presentation, assumed such a background in the reader.

THE SETTING

This program, which originated in a medical setting, is equally appropriate to an in- or outpatient mental health facility or a private office practice. The needed props, materials, and equipment are minimal. The program requires comfortable seating for group members and leaders and, of course, the room must assure privacy and relative quiet. Seating is best arranged in a circle, with sufficient space between people to allow easy eye contact. A classroom arrangement (with the students all facing forward and the teachers at the front of the room) is strongly discouraged.

Although a blackboard or newsprint on an easel would be strongly recommended, they are not necessary. As an alternative to the blackboard or newsprint, materials such as diagrams may be reproduced in advance and handed out. A videotape system (camera, recorder, and TV monitor) can prove helpful (see discussion of sessions 8 through 11, below) but is also not necessary.

NCR (no carbon required) paper is used throughout the program in the Personal Reminder Form and cognitive restructuring homework sheets especially. If unavailable, a photocopying machine or carbon sets can be substituted.

Number of Participants

Eight to twelve is a reasonable number for a group of well-functioning but symptomatic patients. Six to eight patients may be the maximum for a severely depressed group.

Length of Session

Smaller (up to 10 participants) and less symptomatic groups will require only 75- to 90-minute sessions. Larger and more severely symptomatic groups may need up to two hours per session.

Teaching

Through the entire development of this coping skills model of treatment, we have maintained a strong commitment to teaching this method of intervention. We have seen groups entirely composed of health care professionals (nurses, physicians, physician's assistants, and mental health professionals) who became involved so as to learn the techniques for their own personal use as well as to be able to make more appropriate referrals. In addition, we have included professionals who participated in the group in the role of observer/co-leader; we have also had observers who confined themselves to watching from behind a one-way mirror. Each of these techniques can be recommended, depending upon the instructional objective.

A group solely for professionals is highly recommended if they are to be potential referral agents and especially if they have little or no mental health experience. A mixed group of "regular" patients with one or two professionals or students in the role of patient can allow for more teaching of the role of therapist and also allows the mental health professional or trainee to identify with and model both the role of patient and therapist.

Observation behind a one-way mirror constitutes the least involving but also the least intrusive model for teaching. Often students in disciplines other than mental health (e.g., medicine) are exposed to this intervention model as observers behind the mirror. The one-way mirror has proved to be little more than a momentary distractor to patients and allows for a large number of observers.

Fee

Although this program was developed in a prepaid setting, it adapts easily to the fee-for-service model. Preferably a single fee, including all group and individual contacts, would be set for the entire program as prescribed in the manual. Additional contacts, of course, could be arranged, with fees charged as appropriate. The alternative model for fees would be simply to charge for each session attended. We are less enthusiastic about this alternative because it may seem to allow for missed appointments, which would then hinder the treatment's effectiveness.

THE MODULES

The coping skills program consists of four modules or skills, which are taught to the patients in the course of the 15 sessions.

The Relaxation Module (Sessions 1 and 2)

In this module the therapists seek to teach the participant two basic approaches for relaxation: Benson's (1975) Relaxation Response (BRR) and Jacobson's (1938) Progressive Muscle Relaxation (Deep Muscle Relaxation, DMR).

The Cognitive Restructuring Module (Sessions 3 through 6)

In this module the therapists seek to teach the patient alternative ways of thinking as a means of combating mood problems (depression, anxiety, etc.) and behavioral disorders (phobias, substance abuse, etc.). Dysfunctional or distorted patterns of thinking are identified and participants are taught methods of challenging and changing negative automatic thoughts (ATs) and replacing them with more rational responses (RRs).

The Assertion-Training Module (Sessions 8 through 11)

Assertiveness training is a method for supporting more effective interpersonal functioning in the patient who is either too passive or too aggressive. It has a behavioral emphasis that builds on the cognitive skills developed in the previous module.

The Problem-Solving Module (Sessions 12 and 13)

Problem solving teaches the participants how to think about and tackle problems that might otherwise lead to disorders of a cognitive (e.g., dysphoria) or behavioral (e.g., paralysis) kind. It systematizes an approach to dealing with both everyday problems as well as others that are more severe.

CASE ILLUSTRATION

What follows is a case example:

> Ms. M. is a married 36-year-old secretary working for the government who feels unappreciated and discriminated against in her work. She believes that her supervisor treats her unfairly because of her race, giving her more work and less recognition than the other secretaries in the office. She experiences daily periods of depression and occasional (once every week or two) angry outbursts against her co-workers, which she associates with times of extreme tension. She feels that she will never get ahead in her job and will always be pushed aside when it comes to financial or other recognition from her supervisor. She has recently begun to feel that the job is simply

too much and that she cannot handle the psychological and physical experience of the job-related stress. Ms. M. has begun to awaken many mornings with mandibular pain, which her dentist ascribes to bruxism. She (the dentist) has also found some evidence of teeth grinding on the biting surfaces of Ms. M's teeth. Most recently, Ms. M. has been getting headaches on weekday afternoons shortly before leaving work; she describes this pain as a throbbing sensation in the back of her neck. She readily acknowledges that this is a work-related ailment.

Ms. M. was referred by her dentist for treatment in the coping

TABLE 1. Case Illustration of Personalization of Multimodule Approach: The Case of Ms. M.

Problem	Intervention (module)	Goal
Depression	Cognitive restructuring	Alter ATs, substitute RRs about not ever getting ahead.
Angry outbursts	Cognitive restructuring	As above.
	Assertion	Confront supervisor about unfairness, lack of recognition.
Job stress	Relaxation	Use Benson and DMR techniques when feeling overwhelmed.
	Cognitive restructuring	Alter ATs about unfairness of office work distribution.
	Assertion	Confront supervisor about being overworked.
	Problem solving	Job-searching strategies.
Bruxism	Relaxation	DMR for musculoskeletal tension before sleep.
Headaches	Relaxation	DMR.

skills program. The presenting problem—the mandibular pain and bruxism—were addressed in the relaxation module, as was her recent problem with headaches and the overall issue of job-related stress. The second module, cognitive restructuring, was also used to defuse the job stresses and to ameliorate the mood (i.e., anxiety and depression) problems. Difficulties with her boss and co-workers were treated in the assertion module; finding ways to get recognition, job advancement, and—ultimately—find a new position were part of the problem-solving module.

Ms. M. responded well to the interventions. She eagerly participated in the group sessions and was scrupulous in performing the homework assignments. No further treatment was considered appropriate by either Ms. M. or her co-therapists. A six-month postgroup follow-up call found that Ms. M. was still in her job but that she was feeling more appreciated, having gotten a small promotion within the office structure. Her headaches had stopped, as had the morning jaw pain. Her dentist was pleased that there seemed little further evidence of the wearing of tooth surfaces.

THE SEQUENCE

The progression from relaxation to cognitive restructuring, assertiveness, and problem solving in the coping skills program is appropriate both from a pedagogical and a logical stance. Pedagogically, the module sequence progresses from those skills that are least difficult to teach to those that are most difficult. Logically, the sequence follows a building-block approach in moving from simpler to more complex self-help skills that actually call upon the techniques learned in earlier modules.

BIBLIOTHERAPY

The cognitive restructuring and assertion training modules rely heavily on two books: Burn 's *Feeling Good* (1980) and Smith's *When I Say No I Feel Guilty* (1975), respectively. The utility of these books should not be underestimated, nor should they be presented as "optional" to the participants. Surely, both these self-help skills, cognitive restructuring and assertiveness training, can be taught without relying on the books, but only at enormous cost in time and effort. Burns's book, especially, is unique in its ability to translate cognitive restructuring concepts into an easily readable, palatable format. We think of it as being the quintessential example of self-help books because, although it teaches and encourages the reader to work on the issues of therapy, it does not counsel a total do-it-yourself model that might undercut the efforts of the therapist or discourage readers who find they need more than bibliotherapy.

RESEARCH

Our research at the Medical Center was conducted with a symptomatic population randomly assigned to group and individual cognitive behavior therapy (CBT) and traditional group therapy (Shaffer, Shapiro, Sank, Coghlan, 1981; Shapiro, Shaffer, Sank & Coghlan, 1981; Shaffer, Sank, Shapiro & Donovan, 1982; Shapiro, Sank, Shaffer & Donovan, 1982). As of the 12-month follow-up, clinically significant treatment effects for anxiety and depression were maintained for both the individual CBT and for this group model CBT but not for the traditional (interpersonal) group therapy condition.

We have not yet obtained data supporting the effectiveness of this program as primary prevention for nonsymptomatic populations or tertiary treatment for severely symptomatic patients. Therefore, a logical next step in our own research will be to extend the boundaries of our investigation to the treatment of patients who are nonsymptomatic (primary prevention, patient education) as well as severely or chronically symptomatic. In the absence of such data, we would nonetheless recommend the application of this program to the area of primary prevention (i.e., the teaching of these skills to populations "at risk," who have been through significant life stresses and might later become symptomatic—for example, singles new to the geographical area, new parents, people going through work interruption or work change, the newly divorced or separated). With those patients who are severely or chronically symptomatic, we would urge greater caution in the use of this program. This would include careful monitoring of functioning and the ready availability of concurrent treatment or support on an individual basis.

This manual originated simply as a means of reducing preparation time of our successive repetitions and revisions for our coping skills group. It later developed as a means of teaching this program to fellow staff members who could not observe the groups at first hand. In addition, invitations to give workshops on our group program to various community agencies helped encourage us to commit more and more of our ideas to a written format for the sake of consistency and efficiency. Finally, our research—measuring the therapeutic efficacy of our group program—required the standardization of our treatment procedures.

This, in turn, called for yet another level of detail in the reporting and recording of our coping skills program. Thus, through a long series of revisions and amplifications, this manual has become what it is today.

Style

We have reluctantly adopted the exclusive use of the male pronoun in referring to an ambiguous individual, either therapist or patient. We have chosen this third-person referent for convenience in writing and simplicity in reading.

Acknowledgments

We wish to express our great debt to Aaron Beck and Albert Ellis, two theoretical giants in the field of cognitive behavior therapy. The medical practitioners of the George Washington University Health Plan provided an endless flow of patients for our groups; without them, there would have been no practical means of testing out our model. Our colleague Donna Coghlan Donovan was central to the empirical investigation of this treatment approach. Susan Stout, our administrative assistant, provided limitless support every step of the way and deserves no small measure of credit for this product.

1

COPING SKILLS TRAINING AND COGNITIVE BEHAVIOR THERAPY

Thomas L. McKain
Catholic University of America

The coping skills group described in this volume is a form of brief, structured group psychotherapy in which clients are taught a variety of cognitive behavior techniques to be used for reducing both anxiety and depression and for coping more effectively with the problems and stresses of everyday life. The cognitive behavior techniques incorporated into the program (cognitive restructuring, problem solving, relaxation, and assertiveness training) have been carefully chosen to provide clients with a complementary set of coping strategies on which they can draw in dealing with current problems and with a broad range of potential future problems. The program is therefore in a very real sense preventive as well as remedial.

The primary purpose of this chapter is to trace some of the historical roots of the coping skills training approach in cognitive behavior therapy. In addition, two important characteristics of coping skills training are considered briefly at the beginning of the chapter: (1) the "coping" versus the "mastery" model of psychological intervention and (2) the psychoeducational approach. The chapter concludes with a brief consideration of the use of groups in cognitive behavior therapy and of the effectiveness of coping skills training.

THE COPING MODEL

The term used by the authors to identify their program—*coping skills training*—points to significant assumptions underlying their approach. One of the most important of these is that the teaching of effective coping strategies is a more appropriate and realistic goal for psychotherapists than the complete elimination of clients' psychological problems. Although this latter goal seems obviously untenable when stated so explicitly, it is nonetheless ubiquitous in the mental health field (Cummings & VandenBos, 1979). Barrios and Shigetomi (1979) refer to this latter approach as the "mastery" as opposed to the "coping" model of psychological intervention; Cummings and VandenBos have dubbed it "the ultimate cure." In challenging this approach, Cummings and VandenBos state: "We usually act as if contact with a professional psychologist is for a single, simple, unified problem and that six sessions will solve everything forever. No other field of health care holds this conceptualization of treatment outcome" (p. 433).

In developing their program, the current authors have clearly opted for the coping rather than the mastery model. In doing so they have allied themselves with an important trend in cognitive behavior therapy—a trend toward "teaching the client general strategies that can be applied not only to [his or her] current problems but also to difficulties that may crop up in the future, thereby training the client to become his or her [own] counselor" (Chambless & Goldstein, 1979, p. 234).

THE PSYCHOEDUCATIONAL MODEL

The authors have also identified themselves with another important trend in cognitive behavior therapy—the *psychoeducational* approach to the delivery of mental health care services. As Upper and Ross (1980) comment in their book *Behavioral Group Therapy,*

> an important recent development in contemporary psychotherapy [is] the integration of purely educational procedures (such as structured curricula and lesson plans, didactic teaching, and formal exercises) and psychological techniques (such as modeling, behavioral rehearsal, feedback, and reinforcement) into psychoeducational skills training program. (p. 1)

As long ago as the early 1970s, Guerney, Stollack, and Guerney (1970, 1971) strongly argued for the adoption of a psychoeducational model—one in which clients would be taught a variety of coping skills for dealing with current and future problems. The most complete early statement of this psychoeducational model is a 1975 article by Authier, Gustafson, Guerney, and Kasdorf. The most salient feature of the psychoeducational model as those authors define it is its opposition to the traditional medical model of "psychopathology" and psychotherapy. Advocates of the psychoeducational model see their function "not in terms of abnormality–diagnosis–prescription–therapy–cure" (Authier *et al.*, 1975, p. 31) but in terms of "the teaching of personal and interpersonal attitudes and skills which the individual can apply to solve present and future psychological problems and to enhance his satisfaction with life" (Guerney *et al.*, 1971, p. 277).

In many ways the role of the psychotherapist working within a psychoeducational model is analogous to that of the teacher. Clients in psychoeducational psychotherapy "are viewed and treated as students capable of *learning* and *applying the skills taught* . . . and not as patients whose symptoms need to be removed by an expert healer" (Brown, 1980, p. 340; italics added). What sets the psychotherapist teaching coping skills apart from the typical classroom teacher, of course, is the "affective–behavioral–interpersonal nature of what he teaches" (Authier *et al.*, 1975, p. 32).

In a qualified defense of the medical model, Guerney *et al.* (1971) are careful to point out that they are referring to "nonpsychotic" behavior when they recommend a psychoeducational approach; and Authier *et al.* (1975) emphasize that they do not consider the medical model inappropriate "for treating psychiatric problems that have a true organic base" (p. 32). But with these qualifications in mind, Authier *et al.* and Guerney *et al.* urge abandoning the medical model and, in the words of Hilgard, Atkinson, and Atkinson (1975), focusing "on the very practical problems of how people can change their behavior to cope more satisfactorily with the problems of life" (p. 509).

THE ORIGINS OF COPING SKILLS TRAINING

The history proper of the coping skills approach begins with the rapid development in the 1950s of the two systems of psychotherapy from which coping skills training grew: cognitive therapy and behavior therapy. The basic assumption underlying a coping skills training model, however, goes back to Freud and his belief that maladaptive behavior is in most cases a result of life experience or past learning rather than "instinct," as McDougall (1923) held, or genetic factors, as Galton (1883) proposed. Authier *et al.* (1975) comment that "when one considers how long ago this controversy was settled in the minds of psychologists, it seems more difficult to explain why psychologists . . . failed for so long to model themselves after teachers than it is to explain why they are now beginning to do so" (p. 33).

Freud also on occasion described the therapist as an educator and said that the patient should be educable; nonetheless, his views on the "nature of the learning process and the ways in which the patient can be retaught new ways of functioning" differ dramatically from the views of the cognitive behavior therapist (Goldfried & Davison, 1976, p. 15).

Authier et al. (1975) single out Carl Rogers as the first important figure in moving therapists away from the medical model that had dominated the field of psychotherapy since Freud. Rogers's insistence on referring to people in therapy as "clients" instead of "patients" was one aspect of this new point of view. In addition, Rogers (1951) emphasized two ideas essential to the coping skills model in cognitive behavior therapy. First, Rogers felt that it is counterproductive to try to make all the connections between clients' current problems and their past; in his view, it is more important to focus on current problems and attitudes. Second, Rogers believed that clients have the capacity for self-direction and for dealing constructively with their problems. This, of course, is one of the primary assumptions of the coping skills model.

The coping skills therapist differs from Rogers with regard to the best way of helping clients to deal constructively with their problems. For Rogers, the important function of the therapist is to provide an interpersonal environment in which clients can begin to experience their own sense of worth and significance. Within this environment clients can, through talk, begin to gain understanding of the nature of their problems. Under these conditions, Rogers believed, the clients' own capacity for growth will be unblocked and they can begin, in effect, to become their own therapists. For the coping skills therapist, on the other hand, the best way to assist clients to grow and to become their own counselors is to give them an understanding of and competence in using specific, effective techniques for changing their behavior.

Cognitive Therapy and Coping Skills Training

Coping skills training and cognitive behavior therapy both evolved when Albert Ellis (1957, 1958, 1962) and Aaron Beck (1963, 1970, 1971, 1976) came to view the cognitive processes of clients and the identification of these processes as crucial to therapeutic progress. Ellis called his system rational–emotive therapy (RET), and Beck termed his evolving therapeutic model cognitive therapy. The ideas of both of these pioneers form the basis of the cognitive restructuring component of the coping skills program set forth in this volume.

Although behavior therapy was itself just being developed at this time (Wolpe & Lazarus, 1966), RET and cognitive therapy made use of many behavioral techniques (e.g., homework assignments, behavior rehearsal, self-monitoring) which became part of the armamentaria of both behavior therapy and coping skills training (Ellis & Harper, 1975; Beck, Rush, Shaw, & Emery, 1979).

Before considering the history of the coping skills model in cognitive therapy, it is worth mentioning some of the terms which, at times, are used as if they were synonymous with cognitive therapy and with each other and which, at other times, refer to a specific variation of cognitive therapy. Among these terms are *cognitive restructuring, rational restructuring, systematic rational restructuring, semantic therapy, rational behavior training, rational psychotherapy, cognitive therapy, and rational-emotive therapy.* In this chapter the terms *cognitive therapy, cognitive behavior therapy,* and *cognitive restructuring* will be used except when the approach of a particular theorist is being discussed. In its broadest sense, the term *cognitive therapy* encompasses not only techniques such as cognitive restructuring (i.e., techniques that attempt to discover and change those cognitions associated with psychological distress or maladaptive behavior) but also such techniques as problem solving (D'Zurilla & Goldfried, 1971; Mahoney, 1977). *Cognitive behavior therapy* combines these cognitive techniques with more behavioral techniques such as relaxation training, assertiveness training, and the self-control techniques of self-monitoring and self-reinforcement.

From the beginning, Ellis's RET reflected a coping skills training approach, with Ellis emphasizing the educational aspects of his approach (e.g., teaching clients self-help skills which they can apply in solving their own problems). Beck also has stressed much that is important to a coping skills model, including the use of a psychoeducational approach (1970), respecting the capacity of clients to be their own therapists, and providing clients with skills which they can use in dealing with future as well as current problems (1976).

Proponents of other variations of cognitive therapy have also seen their techniques as coping skills to be taught to clients. For example, Goldfried and Goldfried (1975) have stated that the goal of their "systematic rational restructuring is to teach this technique to the client himself, so that once he terminates treatment, he can cope with upsetting situations on his own" (p. 115).

Behavior Therapy and Coping Skills Training

Although the roots of behavior therapy can be traced back to such innovators as Pavlov, Thorndike, and Watson, its major development began in the 1950s with the work of Skinner (1953), Lindsley (Lindsley & Skinner, 1954), Wolpe (1958), and Lazarus (1958). Unlike that of Beck and Ellis, however, the approach of the early behavior therapists did not fit into a coping skills or psychoeducational model. As Guerney *et al.* stated in 1971, "The behaviorists *have* adopted a new theory and new methods of treating people with problems, but in terms of methods of *delivery of service* (i.e., individually oriented diagnosis and prescription) they generally do so within the medical practitioner model" (p. 276). This point of view was reflected by Wolpe and Lazarus in their book *Behavior Therapy Techniques* (1966): "One result of realizing that neurotic behavior is learned is to place the responsibility for the patient's recovery unequivocally in the hands of the therapist, just as in other branches of therapeutic practice, and the patient should know this" (p. 20).

Cautela (1969) was one of the first to argue that behavior therapists should teach clients active skills that could be broadly applied. Cautela wrote that

> the behavior therapist has not, to any extent, attempted to make the individual less susceptible to the development of further maladaptive behaviors; neither has he provided means for the individual to eliminate any such maladaptive behavior without the aid of the therapist. For the most part, the behavior therapist has concentrated exclusively on removing the maladaptive behavior present in the individual when he comes for treatment. (p. 323)

Nevertheless, early behavior therapy had a number of characteristics which pointed in the direction of the psychoeducational coping skills model. Foremost among these was the behavior therapist's view that "psychopathology" is a result of faulty learning (Bandura, 1969; Kanfer & Phillips, 1970; Lazarus, 1971). To the behavior therapist, the client's psychological problems result from the fact that either the person has "failed to learn the necessary behavior" or has "learned ineffective or maladaptive habits" (Hilgard *et al.*, 1975). The behavior therapist thus saw the client as a learner (Authier *et al.*, 1975) to whom new and more adaptive behavior could be taught through the use of techniques stemming from experimentally derived principles of learning. The goal of the behavior therapist, in short, was to provide the client with new learning experiences (Goldfried & Davison, 1976).

This orientation, and its relation to the psychoeducational coping skills model, is summed up by Thoresen and Mahoney (1974): "A major contribution of behavioral approaches to therapy has been the emphasis on teaching and learning, viewing therapy as an educational process in which the client is assisted in learning more appropriate behavior" (p. 142).

A second characteristic of early behavior therapy that appears to endorse a psychoeducational approach was the extensive use of coaching and detailed instructions in the course of therapy (Beck, 1970). This is similar to the approach of cognitive behavior therapists and in contrast to the psychodynamic approach. Wolpe and Lazarus (1966) give an example of these didactic elements in their description of systematic desensitization: "The patient . . . is . . . introduced to the practice of behavior therapy. This is done by means of short didactic speeches, or else in the course of running discussions between patient and therapist . . ." (p. 17).

A third characteristic was the belief—put forward even more forcefully by behavior therapists than by client-centered therapists—that it is a waste of time for the therapist and client to try to establish all the connections between current problems and past history—not because the connections are not there but because, in the behavior therapist's view, these past events no longer function to *maintain* the maladaptive behavior (Goldfried & Davison, 1976). Behavior therapists felt strongly that their time could be better spent trying to help clients acquire new and more successful ways of behaving.

The Shift in Behavior Therapy

By the late 1970s a considerable shift had become apparent in the approach of behavior therapists. This was noted in 1979 by Barrios and Shigetomi and in 1977 by Meichenbaum, who wrote:

> Behavior therapy is shifting from an emphasis on discrete, situation-specific responses and problem-specific procedures to a concern with coping skills that can be applied across response modalities, situations, and problems. For example, instead of viewing systematic desensitization as a therapy procedure designed to counter-condition separately each of the client's fears, one can view it as an instance in which a client learns a set of coping skills that be applied across a number of fearful situations. (p. 144)

How and why did this change take place? Several names stand out in this regard. For example, in the mid 1960s Kanfer and Phillips (1970) developed what they called "instigation therapy," an approach in which the therapist acts as an instigator or motivator to help the client begin a change program but in which the responsibility for carrying out the program is given to the client. As Authier *et al.* (1975) point out, "The advantage of the therapist operating in this role is that it puts the burden of change with the person most likely to be in the best position to assess which behaviors need to be changed: the patient" (p. 39).

At about the same time Cautela (1966, 1967) was writing about a process he termed "covert sensitization," a form of aversive imagery therapy. According to Thoresen and Mahoney (1974), "this procedure was pioneered by Lazarus (1958), who asked a hypnotized client to imagine himself performing an undesired behavior . . . and experiencing aversive consequences" (p. 120). The advantage of covert sensitization was that it could be taught to the client, who could then use it outside of the therapy session as a self-control procedure (Authier *et al.*, 1975).

In 1969, the year in which he recommended that therapists move in the direction of teaching self-help skills to clients, Cautela also put forward a self-control version of desensitization in which the client was carefully taught the procedures involved and was asked to practice the procedures at home. In this year other writers also suggested that therapists become more involved in teaching skills that could be generalized. Krumboltz and Thoresen (1969), for example, suggested that it might be better to teach clients either general strategies for controlling problem behavior, or perhaps problem-solving skills, rather than treating specific problems or symptoms.

What were the reasons for this shift in interest from an approach in which the therapist tried to assume full control of his or her client to one in which clients were being taught skills which they could use in dealing with problems on their own? Barrios and Shigetomi (1979) suggest that one reason may have been the shortcomings of traditional methods such as desensitization and modeling procedures, particularly the fact that results often failed to generalize from the targeted behavior or situation to other problem areas in the client's life. This view was also put forward by Meichenbaum (1977), who stated that "it was mainly in attempting to enhance treatment generalization that a number of investigators developed therapy procedures concerned with skills training" (p. 145).

An increasing interest in prevention may also have contributed to the shift. Cautela (1969), Goldfried and Merbaum (1973), and Meichenbaum (1973) all recommended that clients be taught active, generalizable skills in the interest of preventive mental health (Barrios & Shigetomi, 1979). And as Authier *et al.* (1975) point out, preventive measures in mental health are psychoeducational almost by definition, requiring that clients be instructed in ways of dealing with future problems rather than merely being treated for existing ones. Also at this time there was an increasing realization that, as Miller (1969) pointed out in his presidential address to the American Psychological Association, there were simply not enough providers of psychotherapeutic services to meet the need. To help solve this problem, Miller suggested that people would have to be trained to "be their own psychologists and [to] make their own application of the principles that [psychologists] establish." This view was recently echoed by Barrios and Shigetomi (1979), who stated that "the epidemiological data on anxiety reactions and phobic disorders provide additional justification for coping-skills training programs. Large segments of the general population suffer from performance-debilitating anxiety reactions" (p. 493). In their view, coping skills training has the potential to "maximize preventive effects, reduce multiple anxiety reactions, and minimize treatment duration" (p. 493). The trend toward brief psychotherapy, an approach which has received empirical support (Cummings & VandenBos, 1979), also lends support to this approach.

One of the most intriguing possibilities for the profession's shift in interest to coping skills training is suggested by Goldfried (1977) in a discussion of systematic desensitization. Goldfried writes that

> behavior therapists have . . . noted that, even when they have presented desensitization as a counter-conditioning procedure for the elimination of specific fears, clients frequently interpret the beneficial effects as being due to having learned a strategy for coping with stress in general. (p. 83)

Goldfried cites a study by Sherman (1972), who found that "subjects desensitized to fear of water indicated that their ability to relax helped them in such diverse situations as test-taking, speech-giving, and sleeping at night" (p. 83). In other words, clients were themselves converting the techniques they had learned in behavior therapy into coping skills and applying these techniques to a variety of problem areas in their lives.

This finding is consistent with the experimental evidence indicating that people can be trained to act as their own change agents (Kanfer, 1977; Brown, 1980). Beck (1976) has argued that psychotherapists have underestimated their clients for too long and that they should make better use of their clients' abilities.

Behavior therapists' growing interest in coping skills training also coincides with a revision in these therapists' frame of reference to include cognitive factors. Indeed, Barrios and Shigetomi (1979) specifically cite this as one of the factors responsible for the behavior therapist's growing interest in coping skills training. An important figure in this regard was Bandura, who helped provide the theoretical foundation for the behaviorist interest in cognitive factors, self-control, and self-direction (Bandura, 1969).

It is important to note that there are also certain factors working against the adoption of a psychoeducational or coping skills approach.

Authier *et al.* (1975) point out the difficulty that many therapists have in forsaking the familiar doctor–patient roles associated with the medical model. These are roles that have accorded the psychotherapist a considerable amount of prestige and power. In addition, there is the matter of reimbursement for psychological services by third-party payers. Insurance companies have sometimes refused to pay for psychotherapeutic services that appear to be "educational" in nature. One cannot underestimate the potential power of economics in maintaining support for the medical model and keeping therapists from adopting the coping skills or psychoeducational model.

A VARIETY OF COPING SKILLS TECHNIQUES FOR THE CLIENT

By 1975 Authier *et al.* had observed the trend toward the development of modular units in psychoeducational skills training, with each module devoted to teaching a different coping skills technique. For example, in 1969 Cautela proposed teaching clients five coping or self-control skills: relaxation, desensitization, thought stopping, covert sensitization, and assertiveness. In his chapter on self-management methods in the book *Helping People Change* (Kanfer & Goldstein, 1975), Kanfer included the techniques of anxiety management, self-directed desensitization, and systematic rational restructuring, also recommending the use of such auxiliary tools as contracts, homework assignments, and self-monitoring.

In 1977 Meichenbaum listed what he saw as "certain common treatment components" underlying the many different coping skills programs. These common characteristics included problem solving, cognitive restructuring, relaxation training, and the use of didactic presentation, guided self-discovery, modeling, behavior rehearsal, and graded behavior assignments. And in a coping skills program in a community mental health center for formerly hospitalized psychiatric patients, Brown (1980) included training in progressive relaxation, anxiety management, social skills, assertiveness, and self-reinforcement.

This movement toward the teaching of a combination of techniques was a response to the realization of the complexity of the coping process (Murphy, 1962; Janis, 1965; Meichenbaum, Turk, & Bernstein, 1975). As Meichenbaum (1977) states, "a complex multifaceted training procedure is employed to teach coping skills. When we consider the nature of the coping response to stress it becomes evident that a varied treatment program is indeed required" (p. 147).

GROUPS

Although they began as individual psychotherapies, both cognitive therapy and behavior therapy have made extensive use of groups; even early in coping skills training the group seems to have been the rule rather than the exception (Authier *et al.*, 1975). All group therapies, of course, share the advantages of economy and of showing clients that they are not alone in their problems (Hilgard *et al.*, 1975). Ellis (1977) has listed several additional advantages of a group format for cognitive behavior therapy. The first stems from the educational or didactic nature of cognitive behavior therapy and the fact that explanations and instructions are more easily given to clients in a group format. The second advantage is that, as cognitive behavior therapy requires that clients be made aware of maladaptive cognitions, the therapist can be aided by comments and suggestions from group members. Finally, certain auxiliary behavioral techniques used in cognitive behavior therapy, such as behavior rehearsal and risk taking, require a group format.

The first use of groups in behavior therapy was a group desensitization described by Lazarus in 1961. According to Wolpe and Lazarus (1966), this involved simply orthodox desensitization in a group format. Group desensitization was again described by Lazarus in 1968, the year in which Baker, Kahn, and Weis (1968) described group-administered relaxation.

Assertiveness training, one of the components of the coping skills group described in the current volume, is a common element in behavior therapy, cognitive behavior therapy, and coping skills programs. Lange and Jakubowski (1976) give the following reasons for preferring group to individual assertiveness training: (1) the rationale and examples given by other group members for asserting their rights, (2) the opportunity for the display of nonassertive and aggressive behaviors, and (3) the opportunity to practice assertive responses with a variety of people.

Meichenbaum (1975) mentions two of his early studies (Meichenbaum, 1972; Meichenbaum, Gilmore, & Fedoravicius, 1971) in which group cognitive restructuring was found to be "as effective as individual treatment." Meichenbaum adds that the "group treatment proved easier, and more valuable in fostering behavior change." The reason for this, Meichenbaum felt, was that in group treatment "clients could benefit from a group discussion of their faulty thinking styles and self-statements and by the group discussion of the incompatible thoughts and behaviors they must employ to reduce anxiety and change their behavior." Research by the authors of the present volume (Shaffer, Shapiro,

Sank, & Coughlin, 1981) found, similarly, that their group coping skills program was as effective as individual cognitive behavior psychotherapy with moderately depressed and/or anxious clients.

THE EFFECTIVENESS OF COPING SKILLS TRAINING

Meichenbaum (1975) cites several early studies suggesting that a coping procedures model is more effective than mastery models (Wolpin & Raines, 1966; Debus, 1970; Meichenbaum, 1972). Somewhat earlier, a study by Goldfried and Trier (1974) reported that relaxation taught as a coping skill was more effective than traditional relaxation training. In describing the results of this study in 1977, Goldfried reported that subjects in the standard relaxation training group were told that "the training procedure would have the effect of automatically lowering their overall tension level, so that it would be easier for them to deal with a wide variety of anxiety-provoking situations." Subjects in a self-control relaxation condition were told that the purpose of the training procedure was to provide them with a coping skill which they could actively employ in relaxing away tension in a variety of anxiety-provoking situations.

Goldfried found that

> on most of the dependent measures the greatest improvement occurred in the self-control relaxation condition. Furthermore, when subjects were asked during the follow-up to rate their degree of satisfaction with the amount of change they had seen in themselves at that point in time, their responses revealed a striking and highly significant difference in favor of subjects in the self-control relaxation condition. (p. 87)

Encouraging results were also obtained in a study by Brown (1980), one of the few studies to date reporting on the effectiveness of a broad coping skills training program in which clients were taught a variety of techniques. In this study, conducted in a community mental health center, the subjects were 40 previously hospitalized clients who were randomly assigned to either a coping skills training program or a group counseling control condition. Each treatment was for a total of 30 hours. The coping skills program included progressive relaxation (Bernstein & Borkovec, 1973), anxiety management (Suinn & Richardson, 1971), social skills and assertiveness training, and training in self-reinforcement procedures. The group counseling treatment was devoted to analyzing problems with anxiety and interpersonal relations.

Brown describes the coping skills program as follows:

All sessions began with a discussion of homework assignments and a review of each participant's experience in using the skills practiced in earlier sessions. . . . All techniques as well as homework assignments, session plans, and program rationale discussions were detailed in a student's manual given to each participant. . . . Also during the first session an explicit psychoeducational rationale was provided verbally to the students. (p. 341)

The results of the study were summarized by Brown as follows:

Subjects participating in the program reported significantly lower levels of anxiety and fear and significantly higher levels of assertiveness at posttreatment and at the three-month follow up than did the control group. Further, there was some suggestive evidence that these changes may have been clinical meaningful, since a significantly larger percentage of experimental subjects than control subjects scored in the range of a "normal" control group on the anxiety and assertiveness scales at both posttraining testing intervals. (p. 344)

POSSIBLE REASONS FOR THE EFFECTIVENESS OF COPING SKILLS TRAINING

One of the most important characteristics of the coping skills approach is that it teaches clients strategies that they can then use in dealing independently with problems. Particularly if it includes a cognitive restructuring module, the coping skills training program helps clients to understand the sources of many of their problems and also gives them specific tools for dealing with problems and for reducing anxiety or depression. Beck (1976) points out how different this approach is from traditional psychotherapeutic methods in which the client "is led to believe that he can't help himself and must seek out a professional healer when confronted with distress related to everyday problems of living" (p. 9). In the traditional approach, clients may lose confidence in their ability to understand and solve their problems by themselves, feeling instead that their problems are the result of "mysterious forces" beyond their control (Beck, 1976).

This matter of "self-efficacy," as Bandura (1977) labeled it, is extremely important in dealing with depression. Studies on learned helplessness, for example, suggest that depression may be linked to feelings that one has no control over a situation (Seligman, 1975)—that the sources of pain and gratification are beyond one's control. As Hilgard *et al.* (1975) note, "successful treatment [of depression] often depends on getting the individual to realize that his own responses can be instrumental in obtaining gratification" (p. 467). If the analogy with learned helplessness is correct, then a psychotherapeutic process that helps clients acquire skills they can use to gain control over problematic areas of their lives would be extremely valuable. Following this self-efficacy model, Zeiss, Lewinsohn, and Munoz (1979), for example, have suggested that the "essential components of treatments for depression include . . . training in significant self-help skills, focus on independent use of these skills outside of therapy, and attribution of improvement to the client's new skills" (Fleming & Thornton, 1980, p. 652).

Bandura (1977) felt that the cognitive concept of self-efficacy also played a role in the treatment of phobics, in that the clients' expectations of self-efficacy were the key to whether they attempted to cope with anxiety-producing situations. Similarly, Goldfried and Davison cite an early study by Bloom and Broder (1950) suggesting that the individuals are more likely to be successful in solving problems if they have confidence in their ability to cope.

Another possible reason for the effectiveness of coping skills training lies in the paradox that by avoiding certain problems, a person frequently prolongs and intensifies them. For example, a person who always avoids social events because they produce too much anxiety will never have a chance to overcome this fear. Hilgard *et al.* (1975) point out that it is extremely difficult to extinguish avoidance responses for this reason. By offering an alternative to avoidance—direct coping—along with the skills necessary for successful coping, the coping skills therapist can help the individual break this cycle.

Coping skills training tries to assist clients in taking control of their lives. This training attempts to avoid the problem raised by Thoresen and Mahoney (1974) in their critique of traditional therapy. In their view, in traditional treatment the therapist is in control, responsible not only for assessing the problem but also for carrying out the treatment. They cite research by Patterson (1973) suggesting that in this traditional approach treatment results diminish as contact with the therapist diminishes. There are, in traditional therapy, very real limits to how long a therapist can work with a particular client and on the number of problem areas that can be covered. A coping skills training approach, however, can provide clients with psychotherapeutic techniques which they can use indefinitely—and in whichever areas of their lives they choose—without continued or resumed professional contact.

Meichenbaum (1977) provides yet another reason why coping skills training may be particularly effective. His research with test-anxious students indicated that, before training in coping procedures, they viewed physiological arousal prior to an exam as debilitating; after coping skills training, however, they relabeled arousal as "eagerness to demonstrate competence," and viewed the arousal as "facilitative rather than debilitative." Meichenbaum concluded that "following treatment the client's symptoms are cues to cope, to function in spite of anxiety. In this way treatment generalization is built into the therapy package. The client's symptoms become the reminders to use the procedures he has learned in therapy" (p. 12).

CONCLUSION

The program presented in this manual reflects important trends in cognitive behavior therapy—trends toward shorter and more economical interventions and toward a greater use of group, psychoeducational formats. Most important, however, is its reflection of an increasing trend toward providing clients with a complementary set of cognitive and behavioral techniques that they can use in coping with a broad range of problems. By teaching clients how to use the cognitive behavior techniques of cognitive restructuring, problem solving, relaxation, and assertiveness, therapists using this manual are giving their clients a set of skills that can be used long after contact with the therapist has ended.

2

THE SCREENING PROCEDURE

OVERVIEW

Administration of Research Instruments
Preparing the Patient for the Screening Interview
Discussion of the Individual's Symptoms and Problem Areas
Development of Personal Goals for Each Group Module and for the Group
    Experience as a Whole
Description of the Group Experience, Emphasizing its Relevance to the
    Patient's Goals and Problem Areas
Clarification of Questions or Misconceptions about the Group
Explanation of Group Ground Rules
Explanation of Attendance/Performance Record and Contract

INTRODUCTION

The pregroup screening procedure is designed to follow a thorough clinical evaluation. This initial evaluation can be performed by another mental health professional or one of the two group leaders. Often the patients are not self-referred but are referred to the group by professional evaluators. However, one purpose of the screening session is again to assess the appropriateness of each patient for group treatment as well as to introduce the group concept to the patient.

There is a dearth of research in the area of selecting the most appropriate treatment for any individual patient (Bergin & Garfield, 1971). A second evaluation session for selection purposes aids in again determining the amenability of the patient's problems and personal characteristics to group intervention.

In addition, the patient's expectations of therapy have been shown to be significantly related to the outcome of that therapy (Steinmetz, Antonuccio, & Lewinsohn, 1981). Therefore, an individual interview designed to prepare and orient the patient to this particular group modality enhances the probability of a beneficial therapeutic group experience.

One way that the patient is readied for this group experience is by having the therapist describe the type of group sessions the patient will be attending. The group is described as a structured, didactic experience (unlike traditional group treatments) with an emphasis on skills training and homework assignments to reinforce what is being taught.

Next, patients are given the rationale for the group referral as opposed to a referral to individual treatment. The advantages of group treatment are enumerated, with an attempt to personalize each of them for the prospective group member.

Another way in which the pregroup screening readies the patient for treatment is that it gives him a familiarity with at least one of the group leaders. Knowing one of the leaders in advance of the group enables the patient to feel that he already has an advocate in the group and someone to relate to, other than the referring therapist, should he, at some later point, need individual consultation. In addition, at least one of the therapists would have a special knowledge or understanding of the patient, so that if motivation wanes or special problems arise, the patient has an appropriate therapist with whom to speak.

In addition to developing the rapport mentioned above, the pre-screening therapist can help dispel many myths and fears about group treatment. Many patients come to the group with erroneous preconceptions about group therapy in general or about this group in particular. The pregroup session gives the patient a special opportunity to voice misconceptions and to ask questions and to have them responded to fully by the therapist.

In the screening, several methods are used to personalize the group for the individual patient. After a general orientation to this particular type of group therapy, the patient and therapist together arrive at goals for each module. Initially a virtual smorgasbord of potential goals that could reasonably be met in each module can be presented to the patient. This technique can aid the patient in formulating his own goals. In addition, the patient's major presenting problems can be examined and ways in which each module can address these problem areas can be discussed.

The credibility of the group as a personalized treatment approach can be further established by discussing the population for which the group is generally suited. In doing this, the therapist can use his prior knowledge of the patient through notes from the referring providers (when available) and from other materials such as the Pretreatment Questionnaire (PTQ; see Appendix 1). With this material, the screening therapist can emphasize the appropriateness of symptoms and goals that are already known to be experienced or held by the patient for this particular type of treatment.

In addition to the potential benefits for group candidates of participation in the screening session, this procedure also proves very helpful to the therapist. Several examples are listed below:

1. One of the more difficult steps for the therapist starting a new group is entering a room full of strangers who may or may not be feeling positively about embarking upon the group experience. This screening procedure allows the therapist to meet at least half the group members before the first session is held. This head start serves to decrease the anxiety by giving him some prior knowledge of what to expect from at least half the participants. The therapist is also reassured that his co-therapist has the same relationship with all the other group members. The ideal situation would be, of course, for both therapists to interview each patient. However, the present method serves much the same purpose while also ensuring economy in terms of time and expense.

2. It allows the therapist to tailor his subsequent descriptions of and illustrations in the group to the patients' actual problem areas and goals. Being able to specify the group's relevance for each individual patient can enhance patient–therapist rapport and make it easier for the therapist to illustrate convincingly to the patient the appropriateness of this group to his particular concerns.

3. The group screening procedure can increase the candidates' commitment to the group. This commitment can operate on several levels. For one, there is an initial alliance between the patient and the screening co-therapist which is, at least at the outset, stronger than any alliance the patient might feel toward other group members. This alliance can help ward off potential mutinies around issues that may be controversial (e.g., the meeting time). On another level, the patient's increased commitment as a result of the screening enhances the patient's willingness to adhere to the verbal and written contract with the therapist. This contract includes a commitment to (a) attend all 15 sessions, (b) arrive at sessions on time, (c) complete homework assignments, (d) maintain confidentiality, and (e) participate to the best of one's ability.

4. Finally, a major advantage of the pregroup interview is the opportunity it gives the therapist to screen out patients who may not be able

to benefit from the group or who may seriously detract from the experience of other group members. Patients who should be screened out for their own benefit include the following:

1. Those who are significantly more or less intelligent than other group members. (This disparity can prove discouraging to the patient when the leaders gear the group to a significantly different level of intellectual functioning.)
2. Those who are unwilling to see any psychological component in the etiology or maintenance of their problem areas. (Although dubious patients can often be convinced of the merit of psychological intervention, those adamantly opposed to psychological intervention may find it difficult to participate.)
3. Those who lack motivation to work on their problems. (Such motivation to work and change is, in our opinion, one of the most crucial factors for predicting positive therapeutic outcome.)
4. Those who are interested in working only on one very circumscribed area of concern and/or unwilling to discuss that problem area. (Patients who are totally focused on one specific concern may be unresponsive to a more general skills training approach. If, in addition, the problem area is one that the patient is unwilling to disclose—such as a sexual problem or a specific relationship—his participation in the group may be seriously impaired to the point of eliminating the possibility of any significant gains.)
5. Those who are under such severe stress that they cannot concentrate. (Patients can be anxious and/or depressed to such a degree that they cannot absorb what is being taught in the group. Such a patient may be appropriate for the group at a later time after a few individual sessions and/or after medication has been prescribed.)

Patients who should be screened out for the good of the other group members include the following:

1. Those who are uncontrollably verbose. (Patients who deal with their anxiety by speaking in long monologues and who are not responsive to attempts to limit them often bore other patients and/or lose valuable time for themselves and others.)
2. Those who are experiencing a thought disorder. (A group member who becomes tangential, circumstantial, or exhibits other psychotic manifestations may alarm other group members and/or divert the work of the group.)
3. Those who are vociferously and persistently negative and adver-

sarial. (Patients who criticize many functions and procedures of the group and regularly argue with the therapists on multiple issues consume precious group time, decrease the comfort level of the therapists, undermine the morale of the other patients, and may lead other group members to be less cooperative as well.)

As can be seen, the pregroup screening session is a valuable component of the total group program and can have an effect that pervades the remainder of the treatment. The following is a more detailed description of the screening interview itself, including specific suggestions on conducting the interview proper.

PATIENT SELECTION

The traditional referral sources for outpatient psychotherapy candidates are relied upon for the nucleus of the coping skills group. These sources include self-referral, other psychotherapists, and community agencies (community mental health centers, mental health clinics, and specialized community services such as hotlines. drug and alcohol services, and crisis intervention services). A greater potential source of patient flow is the medical care provider (physicians and midlevel practitioners such as physician assistants and nurse practitioners). Though the latter area is less traditionally a source of patients for psychotherapists, it nevertheless constitutes a highly appropriate resource once these health care providers are educated as to the potential benefits of this coping skills treatment program to their patients. Increasingly, medical personnel are becoming aware of the range of studies recognizing the cost effectiveness of mental health services (Goldberg, Krantz, & Locke, 1970; Follette & Cummings, 1967; Cummings & Follette, 1968). Such psychological interventions have been shown to reduce the utilization of medical services in the aggregate. The administrators and staff of primary care health facilities—such as health maintenance organizations and medical center departments of medicine and community health—as well as private practitioners (internists, family practitioners and primary care physicians) have an interest in stress reduction as well as the appropriate disposition of patients whose primary symptoms are related to anxiety and depression. The coping skills program is consistent with the movement in health care toward an emphasis on attending to the patient's emotional well-being, since it affects the patient's overall health. Thus, a self-help skill-oriented nonlabeling therapy is in the forefront of modern medicine's effort to gain the patient's involvement in his own health care.

FORMAL EVALUATION OF THE PATIENT

If the patient has been referred to the group leaders by a person outside the mental health profession, a formal evaluation is performed. In this complete evaluation, the nature and severity of the patient's presenting problems, as well as his past history of psychological problems, social history, suitability for intervention, and motivation for change are all reviewed and analyzed. A disposition is made following this evaluation. This disposition may include the coping skills program—either as the single intervention or as part of a larger therapeutic strategy.

Prior to the initial evaluation, a Pretreatment Questionnaire (PTQ; see Appendix 1) is mailed to prospective group members. They are instructed to complete the PTQ and to mail it to the evaluator prior to the evaluative session, so that it may be read prior to that appointment. The responses to this questionnaire serve as a rough screening device that helps the evaluator in several ways. First, it enables the evaluator to determine the degree of urgency of the patient's concerns. Second, the PTQ allows the initial interview to pass quickly from the acquisition of surface information to the troubling and central issues that bring the patient to the interview. Third, the questionnaire allows the evaluator to identify those areas of functioning (and dysfunctioning) that are particularly appropriate for the coping skills group and to gear the interview toward a more extensive exploration of these areas.

When the patient has been specifically referred to the coping skills group by a mental health practitioner, an extensive evaluation need not be performed during the prescreening interview. However, when the referral source is another professional outside the mental health field, a community agency, or the patient himself, one of the prospective group leaders can do the extensive evaluation (with the aid of the PTQ). Following this procedure, a screening interview can be performed by the other group leader. This separation of tasks enables the evaluating therapist to center upon a single task (i.e., general assessment) while allowing the second therapist to focus on the task of preparing the patient for the group. The evaluating therapist also has the opportunity to consult with other professionals, when appropriate, about the disposition prior to recommending group treatment. For the patient, the delay in referral accurately conveys the impression that the recommendation for group treatment has been well thought out, with the patient's needs as the sole consideration.

CONDUCTING THE SCREENING INTERVIEW

Administration of Research Instruments

Should the co-therapists choose to measure the effects of their group treatment program, the most opportune time for pretherapy evaluation is immediately prior to meeting with the screening therapist. It is preferable to assess the patient's self-report of symptomatology before the screening session, because this first contact with one of therapists is the beginning of treatment (Cummings & Follette, 1976) and can have an effect on the patient's mood as well as his expectations for the future. Assessment tools should be carefully selected to measure what the group experience attempts to teach and the areas of patient functioning that it attempts to change. The patient can be requested to arrive 15 to 30 minutes prior to the interview to complete any inventories or any behavioral assessment activities. The assessment procedure can be explained to the patient as a means of "seeing how you are doing before the group begins." Additional explanations may include the fact that you are attempting to improve upon the quality of care that you are providing and therefore need this type of measurement to assess your efforts.

Preparing the Patient for the Screening Interview

Following the administration of any research instruments, the patient is given a brief description of each of the four treatment modules (i.e., relaxation, cognitive restructing, assertion, and problem solving; see Appendix 2), a list of problem areas that can be addressed in each module (see Appendix 3), and a list of potential goals for the group experience in general and for each module in particular (see Appendix 4).

Discussion of the Individual's Symptoms and Problem Areas

Following the opportunity to read a description of the group, the patient is invited into the co-therapist's office to discuss the problems and/or symptoms he is experiencing. The examples of problems and symptoms listed in the group description (Appendixes 1 and 2) serve as prompts for the patient in remembering and verbalizing the issues he wishes to address in therapy. The therapist can begin by asking the patient if any of the problems listed pertain to him. This usually elicits several positive responses, which can be followed by further questioning to obtain a fuller picture of the patient's concerns.

It is recommended that initially the burden be placed upon the prospective group member to convince the therapist why he is an appropriate candidate for the coping skills program. It has been the authors' experience that patients leaving the screening experience feeling as though they've *earned* a place in the group are more apt to comply with the group program and report greater satisfaction with the results.

Development of Personal Goals for Each Group Module and for the Group Experience as a Whole

Once the patient has discussed his problem areas, the therapist requests that he establish goals for each of the four modules and for the group experience as a whole. The potential goals listed in Appendix 4 can serve to help the patient in creating his own specific goals for the group. To aid in this process, the screening therapist can ask questions such as "How would you know you had been helped by the group?" or "What would you have to see changed before therapy would seem unnecessary?"

After discussing each goal with the patient, the therapist can make up a goal list, which can be typed and duplicated (see Appendix 5). One copy can be retained by the therapist for future reference, while the other is given to the group member at the first group session as a reminder of and reference to what he hopes to accomplish in the 15 sessions to follow. The list also can be referred to both at the beginning of each module to focus specifically upon goals for that skill area as well as at other times in the course of the group when it would be useful for a patient to evaluate his/her progress (e.g., midway and final sessions).

Description of the Group Experience, Emphasizing Its Relevance to the Patient's Goals and Problem Areas

Now that the screening therapist has had the opportunity to learn about the patient's particular problems and personal goals, the therapist returns to a description of the group. The therapist incorporates those concerns of the patient into this description, emphasizing those areas/modules which have particular relevance to the patient as well as why the group format is particularly appropriate for meeting the needs of this patient. The intent is to reinforce the patient's decision to join the group and to emphasize the flexibility and personalized nature of the group in format and content.

What follows is a list of advantages intrinsic to the group format as opposed to individual treatment. Not all will necessarily apply to the particular patient, but at least several can be mentioned in an effort to assure the patient of the appropriateness of the referral for him, thus establishing a positive expectancy.

Advantages of a Group Format over Individual Treatment

Vicarious Learning

The group format allows patients to observe other group members using the skills they are being taught. Hearing how other patients employ the self-help techniques can motivate group members and also alert them to areas in their own lives where the new methods can be put into practice. Learning through the experience of others is a valuable adjunct to learning through one's own experience.

Fostering Independence

The group format encourages patients to rely upon each other for support and direction. Rather than fostering dependence on one therapist, as in individual therapy, the group provides an atmosphere of interdependence which is less intense and can more easily be transferred to self-reliance.

Peer Learning

An individual more closely resembling the patient makes a more effective teaching model (Barrios & Shigetomi, 1979). Consequently group members who exhibit the same symptomatology and who are perceived to be coping with and overcoming obstacles provide excellent aids to the therapeutic process. This distinguishes the group member from the model who responds perfectly and fearlessly in the presence of problems (as the therapist is often perceived to behave). Such "coping" role models are less available within the individual treatment model.

Learning through Helping Others

The group treatment model provides the patient with the opportunity to help others in the group. Yalom (1970) lists altruism as a basic curative factor in groups. He explains "patients receive through giving. . . . They offer support, reassurance, suggestions, insight and share similar problems with one another" (p. 13). This creates a therapeutic ambiance providing an emphasis on change.

Having Similar Problems

Weiss (1976) points out that the experience of "being in the same boat," in this case, sharing the same problem as a fellow group member, is therapeutic *per se*. The sense of having symptoms in common with another patient in the group can reduce the sense of isolation and desperation.

Public Commitment

The very act of declaring to another person one's intention to change appears to increase the probability that such a change will occur. In a group, this commitment is even greater because it is declared more publicly—that is, to more people.

Encouragement through Others' Successes

The perception that other group members are meeting with success can be inspirational to the patient, especially when these problem areas are viewed longitudinally by the patient (i.e., with a sense of the past). When the patient is able to view the actual changes in another group member and be part of that change system, hope and positive expectations can follow.

Clarification of Questions or Misconceptions about the Group

The screening therapist now turns his attention to clarifying common misconceptions that are sometimes held about groups. The following is a list of some of these preconceived ideas together with the more realistic descriptions of this particular group therapy:

1. *The touchy-feely myth:* Groups are composed of a series of exercises where participants are compelled to physically and/or mentally disrobe in an Esalen-type encounter group.

   The reality: This coping skills group is dominated at least half the time by a classroom environment where blackboards, reading materials, and worksheets predominate. No one is forced to do or say anything he chooses not to.

2. *The least-expensive, least-effective myth:* Group therapy is only watered down individual therapy and is consequently less effective, takes longer, and is only recommended because it is more lucrative for the fee-for-service therapist (more patients seen per unit of time) or less expensive to accommodate the prepaid setting (HMOs).

   The reality: Group therapy is often the treatment of choice for problems warranting professional intervention. The group format provides opportunities for learning and a forum for change that can make it a better choice than individual therapy. Our own research program (see the Introduction to this volume) indicates that the group format is as efficacious as individual therapy for this moderately anxious, depressed, and unassertive population.

3. *The solitary-use myth:* Group therapy is useful only in treating people who have difficulties relating to others.

   The reality: Group therapy is enormously powerful in treating problems involving relationships. However, the group format can be helpful in treating many other problems as well. This particular group does not emphasize any one problem area in those selected for membership.

4. *The fear-of-being-a-casualty myth:* Groups are renowned for the many individuals who have been hurt by them through vicious interpersonal attacks and the abrogation of responsibility on the part of poorly trained or nonexistent leaders.

   The reality: This type of group is highly structured and does not allow for uninvited criticism or inappropriate self-disclosure. These group leaders are professionally trained and would intervene in the group without hesitation should there by any hint of a problem for a particular group member.

Explanation of Group Ground Rules

The therapist next describes the ground rules of the group to the prospective member, using the Attendance/Performance Record and Contract (Appendix 6). The therapist writes the name of the patient on the A/P sheet and explains the various ground rules and corresponding penalties. The intent behind the refundable deposit (using nominal fees) is to press for adherence when the patient is marginally resistant to compliance. Obviously a small fee will not sway the dedicated recalcitrant.

(The behavioral requirements and corresponding penalties can be found at the bottom of the A/P sheet.)

Writing the patient's name on the A/P sheet is a means of giving an active visual cue to him that he has been accepted into the group program. The behavioral requirements of the patient and an explanation for their inclusion follow.

Attendance

The patient is asked to commit himself to attend all 15 sessions. Emphasis is placed on attending all sessions with the explanation that each session builds upon what has been taught in previous group meetings and that, as the group continues to meet, the members come to count on one another's presence for feedback and support.

Promptness

The patient is also asked to commit himself to arriving promptly for each group session because the therapists wish to avoid delaying the formal beginning of each group session and/or repeating the beginnings of sessions for latecomers. In addition, group members who are prompt feel penalized by either losing group time at the beginning of the session or having to listen to the therapists repeat their opening comments. If the group is not delayed and the therapists do not repeat the initial instructions, then latecomers miss out on an important part of the group (e.g., review of homework assignments or the introduction of a new skill module).

Homework

Our experience has shown that homework is an integral and essential element for an optimal group experience. Many patients have reported that completion of their homework assignments has enhanced their learning of specific skills. Consequently, patients are given assignments at the conclusion of each session. These assignments include reading materials that explicate the concepts and skills of present and future modules, practice of newly taught skills, and completion of written logs or homework sheets that also enhance adherence to new regimens and mastery of new skills. The intent is both to extend what would otherwise be a single weekly meeting into the daily life of the group member and to ensure that new skills are adequately practiced once they are introduced and maintained through the life of the group. In addition, completed homework assignments provide the basics for much of the group content. Consequently, those who do not complete their homework assignments may reduce their potential level of involvement in the group; this can serve to alienate them from the group and vice versa.

Buddy System

The patient is informed that from the outset of the group he will be paired with another randomly selected group member with whom he will agree to be in phone contact each week. Other procedures for assigning "buddies" (e.g., problem similarity, level of intellectual or social functioning) have led to patients' suspicions of and protestation about being prejudged and labeled, hence the use of a random selection procedure. The purpose of this buddy contact is threefold: it serves to remind the patient that he is involved in a program of change that extends beyond the weekly group sessions; it enhances a sense of belonging to the group and a concomitant sense of camaraderie with at least one other group member; and it gives the patient a source (other than the therapist) of support as well as of additional information about the skills, procedures, and assignments relating to the group.

Deposit

Each group member is asked to make a voluntary, fully refundable deposit of $20 prior to beginning the group. Each of the four ground rules above (attendance, punctuality, homework assignments, and contact with buddy) have a dollar value attached as a penalty for noncompliance (see Table 2).

The purpose of the deposit is to encourage greater compliance from

TABLE 2. List of Problem Behaviors and Corresponding Penalties

Problem behavior	Penalty (in dollars)
Nonattendance (without call or prior notice)	10
Nonattendance (called with explanation)	5
Incomplete written homework	2
Incomplete reading homework	2
Did not contact buddy	2
Late to group (no call)	2
Late to group (called)	1
Planned absence or lateness	0

the group member in these four crucial areas. Though the actual penalties are nominal, they have, in our experience, proved useful in obtaining greater compliance from the group member who might be "on the margin." That is, he might be undecided about complying in any one area and a financial penalty, however small, can serve to push him in the desired direction of increased compliance. In their weight-reduction program, Jeffrey, Gerber, Rosenthal, and Lindquist (1983) report more favorable results for group contingencies (monetary rewards for total weight loss of the group) than for the use of individual contracts. (They did not find that the size of the deposit affected results.) In light of this finding, we would suggest that therapists might want to experiment with a group contingency model in which the entire group might benefit from a combined effort (e.g., all members report doing daily relaxation practice for a week).

Confidentiality

The therapist explains that confidentiality is essential for a successful group. Group members need to feel comfortable disclosing details about their lives without concern that these confidences will be repeated elsewhere. However, although all communications between patient and therapist are confidential from both a legal and an ethical standpoint, communications between patients or overheard by patients do not enjoy the same privileged status. Consequently, the patient is asked to give his pledge not to divulge the identities of other group members or to furnish to others any details about the personal lives or communications of others that might serve to identify them. This is not to say that group members may not talk in general terms about their own experiences or the procedures and skills taught in the group. We ask only that group members maintain a certain vagueness so as to protect the privacy of their fellow group members.

Participation

The group member is encouraged to be as active as possible both during the group session and in the intervening week. It has been our experience and that of others (Lieberman, Yalom, & Miles, 1973) that the more active group members receive greater benefit from the group experience. Because of the large didactic component in the group, it is relatively easy for group members to remain passive listeners and observers. Consequently, patients are warned to avoid this potential pitfall.

In emphasizing individual responsibility, the group leader can now suggest that prior to each group session, the patient recall what remains of his problem areas and to what extent his goals have been met. It is also the patient's responsibility to take stock following the group—to determine what changes have occurred and, if this self-assessment has been unsatisfactory, to ask what he could have done on his own behalf during the group meeting (see Appendix 10, the Personal Reminder Form).

The therapist explains that the emphasis on taking responsibility for one's own progress in the group is an outgrowth of the philosophy underlying self-help therapy. The patient is called upon to be his own therapist. With progressively reduced dependence upon the group leaders, he is encouraged to rely upon the new skills taught in the group. The patient is reminded that each of the 15 sessions is designed to address problems and provide the beginnings of potential solutions. There is no expectation that the patient will be "cured" by the conclusion of the group. He is called upon to practice religiously and improve his skill level following the conclusion of the group. Only then might he expect a significant reduction in his problems and a parallel attainment of personal goals.

Explanation of Attendance/Performance Record and Contract

The patient is referred to the A/P sheet (Appendix 6) in this final part of the screening procedure. Its first part provides space for a listing of the times and dates of the 15 group meetings. The patient is asked to fill in the dates of the sessions as they are read off by the therapist/screener. The act of writing these dates serves as a means of obtaining a greater commitment for attendance from the patient (he cannot later claim to have been ignorant as to the specific dates). This process also serves to jog the memories of patients who would not otherwise recognize scheduling conflicts.

The second part of the A/P sheet lists the requirements of attendance, punctuality, homework assignments, and contacts with the assigned buddy. The third part presents the schedule of penalties for noncompliance with the four activities. While stressing the optional quality of this refundable deposit program, the screener also attempts to emphasize its potential value in persuading group members to adhere to the ground rules of compliance. We do not expect that the nominal sum of $1, $2, $5, or even $10 will cause someone to give up a vacation or business trip, but we have found such a penalty helpful in the "marginal" cases, where a gentle nudge could make a difference. Though a nominal financial penalty is surely not likely to ensure compliance when a participant is unwilling, the existence of a financial inconvenience might make compliance a bit more likely. This nudge in the direction of compliance—hence the opportunity to enhance learning of the new coping technique—is the philosophy behind the deposit. If this is satisfactory to the patient, he is asked, following any questions he may have, to sign the contract and to bring the deposit to the first session (unless he prefers to leave it immediately).

Modification of the contract because of extenuating circumstances (e.g., financial, attendance, or punctuality problems) are addressed at this point and accommodated. No mention is made of the particular attendance or compliance of any group member at any group session. This avoids the pitfalls of shaming those who do not comply with requirements, yet the A/P sheet will represent a small positive reinforcement to those who are in compliance. There is no concern about the accuracy of the patient's recording. The forfeiture of money is not a means of extracting money from the patient but simply one of fostering adherence to the therapeutic regimen.

Those monies which are forfeited can be used for some charitable purpose (e.g., a donation to a recognized charity or as a "scholarship" for a patient not otherwise able to afford treatment).

3

THE RELAXATION MODULE – SESSION 1

OVERVIEW

General Orientation
First Warm-up Exercise
Second Warm-up Exercise
Sharing of Individual Goals
Description of the Four Skill Modules and Their Relationship to Members'
   Goals
Attendance/Performance Record (A/P Sheet)
Demonstration and Instruction in Benson's Relaxation Response (BRR)
Homework Assignment
Feedback to Therapists
Personal Reminder Form

Materials Needed:
    1. A/P sheet for each patient (Appendix 6)
    2. Individual Goal Sheets from the screening interview (Appendix 5)
    3. Relaxation Practice Log (Appendix 8)
    4. List of Readings and Suggested Readings (Appendix 9)
    5. Personal Reminder Forms (Appendix 10)
    6. Homework Assignment sheets

INTRODUCTION TO THE RELAXATION MODULE

Sessions 1 and 2 provide the major content of the relaxation module. Additional relaxation material is provided through the next two modules. Relaxation is the first self-help skill to be taught because (1) it allows for rather immediate relief in a potentially highly anxious group of people and (2) the group members are able to remain rather passive while still learning and obtaining positive results. Eventually the intent is to encourage greater activity and participation among group members. But this is a gradual process and not necessary for obtaining maximal benefits during this two-session module.

INTRODUCTION TO SESSION 1

In Session 1 a group of total strangers is acculturated into the group process. The intent is to neither traumatize nor trivialize, to have the group members feel good about the experience without making it seem like pure entertainment. The first warm-up exercise is designed to (1) familiarize each of the members with the others' names, (2) give each of them the opportunity to say something personal about themselves, and (3) encourage group members to address each other by name. The atmosphere is usually lighthearted, with much laughter. The second exercise is more serious, allowing each member to behave *as if* he had a serious problem but was not being held accountable for it. This is the first opportunity to express emotion and to make self-disclosures in a singularly safe environment. The remainder of the session is devoted to teaching Benson's relaxation response, a quickly taught, easily learned model for tension reduction. Thus the patient can leave this initial session—a critical session for raising or dashing expectations—feeling more comfortable about the strangers he has just met, more comfortable about self-disclosure, and more in control of his bodily tension.

SESSION 1

General Orientation

The cotherapists begin by introducing themselves by name, discipline, and position in the agency (if appropriate).

The group can be introduced as follows:

> This is the coping skills group. This type of group experience is also referred to by some as a stress-management program. You have all been referred to this group for a variety of reasons. What we plan to do today is to show you how each of your goals and individual problem areas will be addressed in the sessions to follow.

One of the cotherapists then takes attendance by reading the group members' names from the A/P sheets. (These will be distributed and reexplained after a warm-up exercise.) Group members are given a copy of the day's agenda and an explanation of what will be happening for the remainder of the session. Rationales are given for the two warm-up exercises.

First Warm-up Exercise

Name Game

Each group member is asked to think of an adjective that begins with the first letter of his name and that in some way describes him. Then each is asked to give a brief sentence that explains how this particular adjective was chosen. In addition, they must recall and repeat the adjective and first name of each group member who has already spoken. The following are some examples: (1) "My name is Bill . . . Belligerent Bill, because I have a lot of trouble getting along with people at work." (2) "He's Belligerent Bill. I'm Moody Marcia. Sometimes my depression gets me down and that's why I'm in this group." (3) "He's Belligerent Bill, she's Moody Marcia, and I'm Cheerful Charlie. I chose cheerful because people say I'm always smiling."

This exercise is designed to aid group members in learning and remembering each others names. It also helps the members to learn a bit about each other in a very nonthreatening format. Group cohesion is fostered by members being able, early on, to refer to each other by name as they address one another. Also, the repeating of all the names and adjectives often lends itself to humor and can be an effective ice breaker.

Some patients will avail themselves of the opportunity to self-disclose during this exercise and will give an adjective that describes their mood or a problem that they are experiencing. Others will be reluctant or unwilling to self-disclose in any way at this time. This game may be one of the first indicators of who will be most open early on in the group experience.

Second Warm-up Exercise

Secrets Game

All group members are given identical pens and pieces of paper. Each is asked to write down something about himself that he would be uncomfortable telling his fellow group participants. At the same time, they are told that their "secret" will be kept anonymous but that it will be read by another group member as if it were his own. The group is given three minutes to write. The slips of paper are then collected, placed in a container, and scrambled. Each group member, in turn, chooses one slip of paper and tells the "secret" as if it were his own (i.e., interjecting his feelings and elaborating upon what has been written).

This exercise serves as a successive approximation to actual self-disclosure in the group. Hearing one's "secret" discussed by another often minimizes its "awfulness" to its author and makes him more likely to bring it up on his own or to talk about other similarly difficult topics. In addition, one of the main advantages of groups is the opportunity to learn that others have similar problems and that one is not alone in his symptomatology. This exercise expeditiously demonstrates the commonality of problems that exist among the group members without forcing premature self-disclosure. Knowing what may be bothering others early on in the group experience fosters group cohesion through increased empathy. The overall effect is to make the participants more comfortable with themselves, with each other, and with the idea of being in a group.

Sharing of Individual Goals

The individual goal sheets generated by each group member in collaboration with a group leader during the prescreening interview are distributed. Group members are asked to discuss or simply read off some or all of their goals for each of the modules (relaxation, assertion, etc.). A sample, completed goal sheet is included as Appendix 7. Certain group members may elect to reveal only a subset of their goals for any particular module. While the group leaders encourage openness and the sharing of "secrets" (as in the warm-up exercises), there is no direct pressure on *individual* members to disclose specific goals or details of their lives.

The sharing of personal goals proves to foster group cohesion and a sense, experienced by many group members, that they were not chosen at random to be in the group but that there were similarities in goals and symptomatology. In addition to cohesion, there is the common experience of a therapeutic lift described by Weiss (1976) as "being in the same boat." Also, the therapists are given the opportunity quite deliberately to point out (when this is not spontaneously done by the group members themselves) that there are obvious similarities among the group members in goals and presenting problems.

Description of Four Skill Modules and Their Relationship to Members' Goals

Each of the four modules is described from the perspective of how it addresses some of the specific symptoms or general categories of problems just mentioned by the group members. Emphasis is placed on those problems or problem areas that are more common to the group participants. Also, special emphasis is given to problems of those members who are more ambivalent about the relevance of their concerns to the purpose of the group.

For example, if several patients described problems of delayed onset of sleep, cluster headaches, and low-back pain, the therapists would mention each of these problems as specific target areas for the skills taught in the relaxation module (though they would also be addressed in other modules, but to a lesser extent).

Attendance/Performance Record (A/P Sheet)

A/P sheets (see Appendix 6) with the name of each group member are distributed. The group members are reminded of the ground rules they have agreed to in the screening session and told that the deposit can be collected at the end of the session. Next, the group leaders give the dates for all succeeding sessions. This is an opportunity for group members to make note of any planned absences (e.g., vacations, business trips, etc.). These absences will not be counted as infractions of the contract and will not be penalized.

Group members, then, are instructed in filling out the forms, marking compliance, noncompliance, or not applicable for the expectations listed (attendance, punctuality, etc.) for the day's session.

Demonstration and Instruction in Benson's Relaxation Response (BRR)

The first mode of relaxation training to be taught is described by Benson in his book *The Relaxation Response* (1975), in which he outlines what he believes to be the essence of "transcendental meditation" as well as other meditation techniques. Group members are asked whether or not they have had any prior experience with this technique; those who have are asked to share their experiences briefly.

The members are asked to make themselves comfortable in their chairs and to close their eyes. They are then instructed to pay attention to their breathing, yet to breathe normally. After several seconds of regular breathing (as observed by the therapist), they are asked to say to themselves the word *one* (it is initially spelled out for them, O-N-E) each time they breathe out. The word *one* was chosen by Benson for its neutral value. If, for some patients, it is not neutrally valued, then another monosyllabic word can be chosen.

The group members continue breathing regularly while saying the

word *one* consistently with each exhalation. If they should find themselves thinking of or distracted by intrusive thoughts, they need not
become concerned but merely bring their attention gently back to their
breathing out and saying the word *one*. The group is encouraged to visualize in their mind's eye the word *one* each time they say it to themselves.
One popular image is that of a neon sign lighting up the word *one* as
they say it to themselves. Another is seeing the word as if it were written
on a chalkboard before them.

The instruction to visualize the word *one* can, for some patients,
prove to be a distraction and, therefore, a relaxation inhibitor. For those,
we suggest that they ignore the visualization component.

The group is allowed to meditate for two minutes. The therapist
then asks the group members to count slowly to three and then to open
their eyes. Group members are told not to be concerned if there is an
increase or no appreciable decrease in their level of relaxation during
this first experience, as it is unlikely to bear any relationship to how well
they will be able to learn the techniques. Many factors can contribute to
a less than optimal situation for relaxation, such as (1) the newness of the
technique, (2) the presence of others in the room, (3) self-imposed pressure to remember all the instructions in great detail, and (4) the pressure
to perform.

The importance of practice is then emphasized. As in learning any
new skill (swimming, driving, tennis, typing), practice of the newly
taught skill is essential to its effective utilization. Group members are
urged to practice the BRR at times and in places that are conducive to
relaxation yet not likely to promote sleep. (Falling asleep will not
enhance the experience of a successful practice session, since the realization that that deep state of relaxation was reached is delayed until
awakening.) At least initially, patients are cautioned against putting the
relaxation procedure to the test in stressful situations so as to guard
against a premature trial of this fledgling skill. Only after several weeks
of practice can the skill be useful in stressful situations.

Homework Assignment

(1) Patients are asked to practice the BRR twice daily for five minutes. (2) They are given Relaxation Practice Logs (Appendix 8) on which
to record their practice. They are asked to complete the sections on the
BRR including a notation about that which may have aided or hindered
them in their practice sessions. (3) They are asked to purchase and to read
the first three chapters of *Feeling Good* (see Appendix 9). (4) Buddies are
assigned on a random basis by the therapists and are asked to exchange

phone numbers. Each buddy pair is asked to make one contact between the two of them approximately midway through the seven days between sessions. (5) Homework assignment sheets are handed out.

Feedback to Therapists

Following the homework assignment, group members are asked at the end of each session to volunteer their positive and negative reactions to that day's group experience. They are requested to discuss what they found most helpful in this session and, also, to make suggestions about what they might want to change for future sessions. At least five minutes should be allotted for this agenda item. The group leaders need to be vigilant that the group members do not use this time to continue an earlier discussion or make additional points about the session's content. They can be gently reminded that this time is specifically for feedback to the therapists.

Important information can be gleaned from such a discussion (e.g., the therapists may find out what they could have done differently that day to elicit more voluntary participation). It is also a time when misunderstandings or misperceptions can be clarified (e.g., during later sessions, a patient may state that he feared a fellow group member had been "put on the spot" too much during that session, and the group member in question may then confirm or deny this supposition).

An additional advantage to the feedback session is that it establishes a collaborative relationship between the leaders and participants and forms a sort of co-ownership of the group and its future.

Personal Reminder Form

At the end of each session, each group member is asked to complete the Personal Reminder Form (Appendix 10). On this form, the participant records the number and date of this session, the module being taught, and any skills or insights obtained during this session. In addition, the participants are asked to do some planning of what they would like to get from the following session, both intra-and interpersonally.

This form is designed to aid the group member in concretizing the skills he has gleaned from the group experience during that session and in remembering and internalizing what he has learned about himself and his problem areas.

The additional emphasis on the upcoming session helps the group member to take an active role in planning the progress of his treatment. Often, at the end of the group, a patient may wish he had brought up something that was bothering him or had given some feedback to another group member. These realizations are often lost during the week, and the reminder form can serve to jog one's memory so that the desired goals can be accomplished the following week.

Finally, these forms serve as additional feedback to the therapists on how well the participants are learning and incorporating what is being presented to them each week. (A copy of the form is handed to the therapists by each group member at the conclusion of the session.) A sample completed Personal Reminder Form is shown in Appendix 11.

HOMEWORK ASSIGNMENT—SESSION 1

1. Practice BRR twice daily for five minutes.
2. Record progress doing BRR on Relaxation Practice Log (Appendix 8).
3. Read Chapters 1 through 3 in Burns's *Feeling Good* (see Appendix 9).
4. Have one phone contact with your buddy.

THE RELAXATION MODULE – SESSION 2

OVERVIEW

Distribution of A/P Sheets, Attendance Taking, Review of Homework, and
   Completion of A/P Sheets
Answering Questions about Homework Assignment
Collection of A/P Sheets and Relaxation Practice Logs
Deep Muscle Relaxation
Homework Assignment
Feedback to Therapists
Personal Reminder Form

Materials needed:
   1. A/P Sheet for each patient (Appendix 6)
   2. Relaxation Practice Log (Appendix 8)
   3. Relaxation Sequence with cue words (Appendix 12)
   4. Homework Assignment sheets
   5. Overview of Session 2
   6. Personal Reminder Forms (Appendix 10)

INTRODUCTION TO SESSION 2

Prototype of the Group Session

This session establishes the regular sequence of all subsequent sessions. It begins with the general housekeeping chores of attendance taking, distribution of A/P sheets, reminding the participants of what the exact assignment was, and then the collection of A/P sheets. Time is allotted for replying to questions about the past week's session and homework assignments. Collection of written assignments with some perusal by one of the co-therapists follows. The new material is introduced, including material from past modules, when appropriate. The homework assignment is distributed with the Personal Reminder Form. Finally, the therapists request both positive and negative reactions to the session.

In Session 2, deep muscle relaxation (DMR) is the only new material introduced. Each group session to follow will contain some form of relaxation experience either in the form of new material or review. DMR is the second of two relaxation techniques to which the group members are exposed. It is our experience that the BRR is most useful for a general quieting response and for relief in syndromes involving smooth muscles (e.g., gastrointestinal distress). The DMR has been found particularly useful in those syndromes involving striated musculature (e.g., headache, bruxomania). These clinical findings, however, reflect trends and are not without exception. Consequently, both techniques are taught without reflecting a bias as to which is likely to work better for a particular patient's problem. The patient's own experience is relied upon in determining which technique will be used at which time, and the regular practice of both techniques is urged.

SESSION 2

Distribution of A/P Sheets, Attendance Taking, Review of Homework, and Completion of A/P Sheets

A/P sheets are distributed and attendance is taken immediately at the outset of the session. The homework assignment is reviewed by referring to the Session 1 homework assignment handout.

Answering Questions about Homework Assignment

In reviewing the homework assignment from the last session, questions are encouraged about the relaxation process itself as well as about the use of the Relaxation Practice Log, the buddy system, and details about obtaining the Burns book. (Questions concerning the *content* of the Burns book are deferred until Session 3.)

Collection of A/P Sheets and Relaxation Practice Logs

A/P sheets are collected during this question/answer segment of the session. Relaxation Practice Logs are also collected and perused by one of the group leaders during this sequence. Any glaring errors may be tactfully corrected at this point in the group or at the conclusion of the session for a particular individual.

The following is a list of typical problem areas encountered in Session 2. Included as well are recommendations that could be suggested by the group leaders. Where appropriate case examples are also provided for illustration.

Problem: Incorrectly filling out the Relaxation Log.
Recommendation: It is often helpful to reiterate instructions for the entire group.

Problem: Lacking motivation to practice regularly.
Recommendation: The leaders ask the group member to refer back to his goal sheet and to look at whether the accomplishment of these goals would be worth the effort involved in regular practice. Often an accounting-ledger-sheet format that looks at the advantages and disadvantages of achieving these goals, given the effort involved in reaching them, can assist the patient in "finding" the motivation.

Problem: Though there is an appreciable sense of increased relaxation, the thoughts continue to intrude into the patient's mind.
Recommendation: Often these problems coincide with a misunderstanding of the passive nature of the BRR. The patient is instructed to allow the thoughts to flow in and out of his mind and not to take an active role in their resolution.

Case Example

A patient found that trivial problems intruded when she was doing the BRR (e.g., what clothes to set out for the next day, what time she would set the alarm to ring the next morning). She was instructed to become indifferent to finding the answers to the problems while relaxing. They could easily wait for her to be finished. She was also asked to repeat these instructions to herself during her practice session.

Typical problem areas that would be more appropriately corrected after the session concludes include (a) some indication of a significant exacerbation of pathology (e.g., deepening of a depression); (b) a gross misunderstanding of the instructions, which might lead to a sense of embarrassment; (c) a special communication to the therapist implicitly suggesting a request for a personal reply; or (d) a level of noncompliance possibly suggesting some problems over control and defiance that would best be defused and dealt with in a private setting, perhaps in an individual consultation hour.

Deep Muscle Relaxation

The second relaxation technique is now introduced. DMR's historical roots in the Progressive Muscle Relaxation of Jacobson (1938) are first discussed; it is explained that DMR is a greatly shortened version of the 16-hour training procedure developed by Jacobson. Next, other relaxation techniques are listed and compared as well as contrasted with DMR. These include the BRR (with which all the group is now familiar), Silva Mind Control, Transcendental Meditation, Yoga, self-hypnosis, and Lamaze natural childbirth, among others. The list need not be exhaustive. The intent is to tap into the past experiences of group members, to make this next phase of the relaxation training more familiar, and to engage the group in conversation or the sharing of experience that will be useful in this and future modules.

Heidl and Borkovec (1983) describe the problem of relaxation-induced anxiety where the patient may experience an actual increase in anxiety-related symptoms consequent to engaging in relaxation exercises. Of course, this phenomenon is not described or suggested to patients, but its existence is yet another rationale for presenting two different kinds of relaxation-induction procedures. Heidl and Borkevec report a higher incidence of relaxation-induced anxiety with focused passive process relaxation (e.g., BRR) than with a focused somatic attention procedure (e.g., DMR). Their findings suggest that it is unlikely that both procedures would result in an increase in anxiety.

The leader next describes the uses of DMR and its offshoots. These include general relaxation, relaxation of specific body parts, and as an integral part of such medical and psychological interventions as treatment for various phobic conditions, sexual dysfunction, hypertension, and natural childbirth.

Next, the process of relaxing using DMR is illustrated by one of the co-therapists. In less than 30 seconds, the demonstrator should, with little or no movement, be able to relax his body totally while "taking an inventory" to find and relax any body parts that showed residual tension. This is preceded by the therapist announcing his SUD (Subjective Units of Discomfort) level and then stating his postrelaxation level accompanied by "I'm now appreciably more relaxed." The group is told that an explanation of the SUD concept is to follow shortly. The group is also told that this illustration demonstrates the endpoint of relaxation training and requires several intermediate steps and several weeks of daily practice to achieve.

Before the actual teaching of DMR, the group members are cautioned that any muscle tensing they are instructed to engage in as part of the training will not, and should not, call upon them to exert all their strength. Any temptation to use maximal tensing should be resisted, as it is counterproductive. For those with contact lenses, keeping the eyes shut for extended periods may prove uncomfortable and distracting. Therefore, occasional opening of the eyes would be appropriate. Those with back problems or other orthopedic symptoms should be instructed either to moderate or ignore any instructions to tense these areas.

The SUD Concept

This serves as a means of developing a common language with which to assist the group members in communicating about personal levels of tension. The Subjective Units of Discomfort (SUD) scale (Wolpe & Lazarus, 1966) is introduced. Group members are asked to visualize an equal-interval scale with 100 points, similar to a thermometer. This scale has anchor points of 1 and 100, describing states of total relaxation and total tension respectively. (For some, the first point is the equivalent of being sufficiently relaxed to fall asleep.) The scale is ordinal; that is, each point is equidistant from the next (e.g., the distance between 29 and 30 is the same as that between 86 and 87). Following this explanation, each member is asked, in turn, to give a number describing his current level of subjective tension. It is emphasized that these numerical descriptions are totally subjective and that one member's 25 might be another's 60. The SUD level of each group member is recorded before and after this session's relaxation experience. These figures may be used later by the leaders to screen for patients with difficulties in learning the technique and also may be used daily by the participants as reference points in homework practice sessions.

Teaching DMR

The group leader begins the actual instruction in DMR by reiterating the precautions regarding contact lenses and orthopedic problems. He asks that the group members make themselves as comfortable as possible by loosening any tight or restrictive clothing, uncrossing their limbs, putting anything on their laps on the floor, removing sport coats, loosening ties, removing eyeglasses, and so on. These accommodations for comfort should be purely voluntary. The cost in anxiety to someone wondering whether his feet will smell or eyeglasses will be broken is not likely to be made up for by an increment in relaxation if shoes or glasses were to be removed. Next, the members are asked to keep any extraneous or unnecessary movements to a minimum during this training. They are also asked not to speak or open their eyes (if possible), as this will distract them (and, in some cases, others) from getting the most from the relaxation instructions. If any of the instruction is unclear, the group member is asked to open his eyes and observe either of the two group leaders who will be participating in the relaxation procedure along with the group. (The leader is himself a participant in these exercises, thus relieving the members of the discomfort of being observed while engaging in exercises that might make them feel awkward or foolish.) In addition, the leader has a better idea of how long patients should be allowed to tense certain muscle areas if he is also doing the tensing himself. Participants are reassured that they need not memorize the sequence of the exercise to follow. A handout (Appendix 12) will provide them with this information.

What follows is a script of the DMR exercises from which therapists may read before developing their own personalized versions.

RELAXATION SCRIPT

Part 1

Let's begin by settling down into your chair as comfortably as you can. Close your eyes and try to regulate your breathing. Just be as comfortable and relaxed as you possibly can *(long pause)*.

Now let's start with your nondominant hand. That means if you are right-handed you'd use your left hand, if you are left-handed then you'd use your right hand. With your nondominant hand, make a fist—make it very tight—feel the tension in your fingers, in your hand, even upward into your forearm—feel the tightness and the tension you can create and now *(pause)* relax; let your fingers slowly uncurl and feel the sense of tension drain away. Do that again now *(pause)*; with the same hand make a fist, feel the tightness and tension and relax *(pause)*. Very good.

Now with your other hand, I would like you to make a fist. Make a tight fist, feel the tension *(pause)*, in your hand, your fingers, and *(pause)* relax. Again experience the feeling of tension reduction as your fingers uncurl and feel more relaxed *(long pause)*. Do that again now *(pause)*, with your dominant hand make a fist, feel the tightness *(pause)*, study it *(long pause)*, and relax *(long pause)*. Very good.

Now with both arms I'd like you to, as if there were a string around your fingers, I'd like you to pull your fingers all the way back. That is, beginning with your palms facing downward you'll cause your fingers to gradually point up toward the ceiling. Pull your fingers backward, feeling the tension along the backs of your hands, along your wrists, forearms, feeling the tension you create there *(pause)*; it's with both hands now *(pause)*, experience the tension you can create and now, as if someone had cut the string pulling your fingers back *(pause)*, relax, just let your fingers fall back down *(pause)*, allowing your hand, your wrist, and your forearm to relax. Do that again now *(pause)*, fingers pulled back experiencing the tension along the back of your hand, your wrist, forearm *(pause)*, feel the tension *(pause)*, study it *(pause)*, and relax. The string is cut—fingers, forearms, and wrists all relax *(long pause)*.

Moving upward into your upper arms, I'd like you to flex your biceps as if you were a strong man in the circus—arms bent, hands above your head and flexing the large muscle in your upper arm. Tense your biceps muscles by bending at the elbow, feel the tension in that muscle *(pause)*, create the tension *(pause)*—experience it—*(pause)* study it *(pause)* and relax. Again letting your arms just lie comfortably perhaps in your lap, perhaps on the arm of your chair *(pause)*, just relax. Do that again now. Flex your biceps *(pause)*, feel the tension you can create there *(pause)*, study it, remember what it feels like and now *(pause)* relax *(pause)* and remember what this comfortable state feels like too *(pause)*, noting the contrast between tension and relaxation.

Moving on to the triceps, the muscle that opposes the biceps, I'd like you to tense your triceps muscles by stretching both arms straight out as if you were sleepwalking with your elbows locked *(pause)*, feel the tension you can create there, feel the tension, the tightness, the constriction and *(pause)* relax. Just let your arms drop comfortably, noting the contrast between the tension you had created in your triceps and the current feeling of relaxation *(long pause)*. Do that again now, please. Arms stretched out, elbows locked, triceps tensed, feeling the sense of tightness and *(pause)* relax—again you should be noting the contrast between the tension that you had just created and now this feeling of relaxation. Fingers and hands relaxed *(pause)*, wrist *(pause)*, forearms, now upper arms *(pause)*, all relaxed.

Moving to your shoulders now, I would like you to shrug them. Please push your shoulders all the way up as if they were going to touch your ears *(pause)*—pull them up now *(pause)*—feel the tension you can create *(pause)*—feel the tightness and constriction and *(long pause)* relax. Letting your shoulders droop comfortably—relaxed—the tension drifting away more and more and feeling the relaxation as it radiates through your arms. Shrug your shoulders again now, please. Recreating the sensation of tightness, tension in your shoulders, your neck, your upper back *(pause)*. Study the tension . . . remember how it feels. Now *(pause)* relax. Let the tension drain out of your shoulders, through your upper arms, forearms, out your fingertips, allowing a feeling of comfort, perhaps a sense of warmth and heaviness to flow through your arms.

Moving now to your face, we will be paying particular attention to your forehead, where a lot of tension can result in a headache. What I would like you to do is to wrinkle your brow by raising your eyebrows *(pause)*—wrinkle it—*(pause)*. Feel that tension, study it *(long pause)*, and now smooth out the forehead *(pause)*. Smooth it out, feeling more comfortable—more relaxed *(long pause)*. Note that there is a contrast between the tension you had created and now this current state of relaxation *(long pause)*. Do that again please, but this time I would like you to furrow your brow by bringing your eyebrows together. Feel the furrows in your forehead (if you can't sense that it is furrowed, you can feel it with your hand), try to experience that tension that you can create in your forehead, the muscle that we call the frontalis muscle *(pause)*. Study that tension *(long pause)*, and now smooth it out *(pause)*, smooth it out *(pause)*—experience the difference, that contrast between tension and relaxation *(long pause)*.

Moving down your face we come to your eyes *(pause)*. I'd like you to tighten your eyes as if you were squinting with your eyes closed—feel the tension you can create around your eyes *(long pause)* and relax *(pause)*, eyes just lightly closed *(pause)*, a greater sense of relaxation surrounding your eyes *(long pause)*. Do that again now please—tighten your eyes, real tight *(pause)*—feel the tension you can create *(pause)*, and now relax *(long pause)*. Very good.

Now we come to your mouth, and we'll start with your lips. What I'd like you to do is to purse your lips *(pause)*, as if you were sucking a lemon and feeling that tightness and constriction in your lips *(pause)*. Purse up your lips, feel the tightness surrounding your mouth, especially in the lips *(pause)*. and relax *(long pause)*—with your lips just lightly closed now *(long pause)*. Do that again please. Constriction of your lips, pursed as if you were sucking something sour *(pause)*, study the tension *(pause)*—feel the tightness *(pause)*, and relax, noting the difference between tension and relaxation *(long pause)*. That's fine—now just relax.

As we move inside the mouth now, I'd like you to press your tongue to the roof of your mouth *(pause)*—press it up *(pause)*—feel the tightness and tension you can experience in your tongue *(long pause)* and relax *(pause)*—tongue just resting comfortably in the mouth now *(long pause)*—a greater sense of relaxation *(pause)*. Do that again now, please. Tongue pressed against the roof of your mouth, feeling the tightness, study it *(long pause)*, and relax *(long pause)*.

Now for your jaw *(pause)*—what I'd like you to do is to jut your jaw out *(long pause)*, stick your jaw out *(pause)*, and feel the tension you can create on the back and underside of your jaws *(pause)*. Almost up to your ears you can feel the tightness and constriction you can create by jutting out your jaws *(pause)*—study that tension please *(long pause)* and relax. Very good. Let's do that again now. You're jutting your jaw out, stick it out *(pause)*—feel the tension, very good *(long pause)*, and now relax. Relax comfortably, feeling the contrast now, the sense of relaxation *(long pause)*.

Now we move downward to your throat *(long pause)*. What I'd like you to do, I'd like you to draw in a breath as if you were going to yawn *(pause)*—open your mouth wide, draw in a breath *(pause)*, feel the tightness in your throat *(pause)*—pull in your breath now and feel the constriction *(pause)*. Now you can follow through *(pause)*—just yawn and follow through as if you actually were yawning *(pause)*—noting the contrast—*(pause)* note the sense of relaxation that you feel in contrast to the sense of tightness and constriction that you had just created in your throat. Let's do that again now, please *(pause)*. As if you were to begin to yawn, pull your throat tight *(pause)*—remember this feeling *(long pause)* and relax. Follow through with the yawn, and then relax *(long pause)*. Very good *(long pause)*.

Now we move to your neck, a very common site for one to experience stress. It is also very much involved with the origin of tension headaches, the kinds of headaches you get when you are under psychological stress, when you might feel a tightness in the back of your neck. I'd like you to push your head back, but not so far back as to feel awkward or painful *(pause)*—press your head back *(pause)*—feel the tightness in the back of your neck, your upper back, and shoulders *(pause)*, and now I'd like you to slowly bend your head forward *(pause)*; bring it forward as if you were trying to press your chin against your chest, but do not force it too hard *(long pause)*—feel the tension that way. And now just bring your head into an upright position and feel the sense of relaxation *(long pause)*. Do that again now, please. First, head is pushed back feeling the tension in the back of your neck *(pause)*—study the tension *(pause)*, and now slowly bringing your neck forward, toward your chest *(pause)*—so that you can feel that tension and *(long pause)* relax. Just bring your head to an upright position, feeling comfortable and relaxed *(pause)*, noting the contrast between what you feel now, the sense of relaxation, and that prior sense of tension and constriction.

Next, still concentrating on those feelings in your neck, I'd like you to *slowly* turn your head all the way to the left *(pause)*, turn it all the way to the left, that's good, now slowly, slowly turn it to the right *(long pause)*, all the while studying the tension and slowly bringing your head to a forward position *(pause)*—relax and note the contrast between tension and relaxation *(long pause)*. Do that again, please *(pause)*, now turning your head slowly to the left, feeling the tension *(pause)* and then turning slowly again to the right *(pause)*, again studying the tension *(long pause)*. And now to a forward position—realizing that sense of relaxation coming now to replace the sensation of tension *(pause)*. Just let the relaxation spread, perhaps becoming a feeling of warmth or heaviness through your fingers and hands *(pause)*, wrists *(pause)*, forearms *(pause)*, upper arms *(pause)*, letting it spread through the shoulders *(pause)*, facial muscles, now *(pause)* your scalp and forehead *(pause)*, your eyes *(pause)*, your lips *(pause)*, tongue *(pause)*, your jaw *(pause)*, your throat *(pause)*, and now your neck. More and more relaxed *(pause)*, more and more relaxed.

Moving down to your chest, I'd like you to take in a deep breath *(pause)*, breathe it in *(pause)*, suck in your breath *(long pause)*—feel your chest expand with the tightness *(pause)*—hold the breath now, please *(pause)*—feel the tension and tightness *(pause)*, and now slowly, through your nose and mouth, exhale. That's it *(pause)*. Slowly exhale *(pause)*, feel the tension and the tightness being expelled from your body *(pause)*. When you are ready, take in another deep breath and hold that, too *(pause)*. Feel the tension now, and concentrate on it. And again *(pause)*, slowly exhale through your nose and mouth *(pause)*, feeling the greater sense of relaxation as you simply expel the tension. You can do that again now, please *(pause)*. Pull in a deep breath and *(pause)*, after you've felt the tension *(pause)*, just slowly exhale *(long pause)*. O.K. that's good. And now just continue to breathe evenly and comfortably in a relaxed way, noting the greater sense of relaxation in your chest *(long pause)*. Now I'd like you to push your chest out as if you were standing at attention in the army. Push your chest out as far as it can go *(pause)*—feel the tension you create in your upper back, your shoulders, neck, and in your chest *(pause)*—feel the tension *(pause)*, study it *(pause)*, and relax. Very good *(long pause)*. Do that again, please. Push out your chest, feeling the tension in your upper back *(pause)*, shoulders *(pause)*, and in the back of your neck *(pause)*, study the tension in your chest now *(long pause)*, and relax. Very good *(long pause)*.

Now we move down to your stomach and abdomen. What I'd like you to do is, I'd like you to pull in your stomach as if it were to touch your spine *(pause)*, pull it all the way in *(pause)*, feel the tension you can create there *(pause)*, and then relax *(pause)*. Now push it out *(pause)* and feel the tension you can create that way *(pause)*—that's good *(pause)*—and now relax *(long pause)*. Very good. Just feel the sense of relaxation as it takes over in your stomach and abdomen, your chest, upper arm. Do that again now, please. Pull in your stomach as if it were to touch your spine *(pause)*, and relax *(pause)*. That's it, feel the tension *(pause)*, study it *(pause)*, and relax. Very good. Study the sense of relaxation now as it comes to replace the sense of tension *(long pause)*. This time I'd like you to pull in your stomach, do it again, pull it in *(pause)*, and now I'd like you to make it as hard as you can, as if someone were about to punch you in your stomach; you will want to make it as hard as you can *(pause)*, feel the tightness that you can create that way *(long pause)*, and relax. Very good *(pause)*. Just feel the sense of relaxation that spreads through your trunk, just let the sense of heaviness and warmth spread through your body *(long pause)*.

Now for your lower back, I'd like you to arch your back away from the chair, arch it up feeling the tightness that you can create in the small of your back, and relax *(long pause)*. Just let your back sink into the chair feeling more relaxed now, more and more at ease *(long pause)*. Do that again now, please. Arching your back up, feel the tension you can create, study the tension and relax, feeling the heaviness *(pause)* and the relaxation spreading upward from your lower back *(long pause)*.

Moving lower now, I'd like you to clench your buttocks *(pause)*. Feel the tightness that you can create there *(pause)*, feel the tension, study it *(pause)*, and relax. Very good. Just relax *(long pause)*. Do that again now, please. Clench your buttocks *(pause)*, feel the tightness that you can create *(pause)*, and relax *(pause)*. Very good *(long pause)*.

Now for your legs. I'd like you to stretch your legs straight out, with your knees locked and your toes pointed away from your face *(pause)*. Legs straight out, knees locked, feel the tension you are creating in your calves, in your thighs *(pause)*, feel the tension *(pause)*, both legs straight out *(pause)*, study the tension *(pause)*, and relax. Very good *(long pause)*. Feeling the greater sense of relaxation up and down your entire leg, you'll note that you needn't tense any other part of your body when you tense your legs . . . they're independent of your trunk, your face *(long pause)*.

Let's do that again now, please. Legs straight out, toes pointed away from your face, feel the tightness along the back of your leg, your calf, feel the tension *(pause)*, and relax *(pause)*. Just relax. Let the relaxation spread through your legs . . . radiating through your entire body, the warmth, the heaviness replacing any vestiges of tension that might remain *(long pause)*.

This time I want you to straighten out your legs but with your toes pointed inward toward your face. You will notice the tension created in the backs of your knees, the underside of your thighs, and in your calves. Remember that feeling *(pause)*, and relax *(long pause)*.

Let's do that again now, please. Legs outstretched, feeling your knees locked, your toes pointed toward your face *(pause)*, feel the tension, study it *(pause)*, study the tension on the backs of your knees, your thighs, your calves *(pause)*, and relax *(long pause)*. Just continue relaxing now *(long pause)*.

Now we move down to your feet. I'd like you to curl your toes downward. Feel the tension you can create, on the bottoms of your feet, in your toes, and in your feet in general *(pause)*. Feel the tension *(pause)* and relax *(long pause)*. Do that again now, please. Toes curled downward, study the tension *(pause)* and relax *(long pause)*.

Now I'd like you to tense your toes by curling them in the opposite direction. Curl them upward *(pause)*, have them point toward the top of your body *(pause)*. Feel the tension you can create that way, in the bottoms of your feet again, in your arches, feel the tension *(pause)*, and relax *(long pause)*, Just relax, sensing, enjoying, the reduction in tension. Let's do that again now. Toes curled upward, feeling the tension along the bottoms of your feet, in your feet in general, through your toes, your arches, just feel the tension *(pause)*, and relax *(long pause)*. Just relax *(long pause)*. Very good *(long pause)*.

Part 2

Now what I want to do is to review your whole body with you, and without doing any prior tensing at all, I want you to allow yourself to relax just a bit more to get all the residual tension out of your body *(pause)*. So as

I name the specific body part, just allow the remaining tension to dissipate *(pause)*. You don't have to tense it, I don't want you to even have to move it, just concentrate on letting the tension just drain out of each part of your body *(pause)*. Let a sense of heaviness and warmth replace the sense of tension *(pause)*. So we'll start with your fingers now *(pause)*. Allow them to be more and more relaxed *(pause)*, and your hands *(pause)*, your wrists and forearms, more and more relaxed *(pause)*, upper arms relaxed, biceps and triceps, becoming more comfortable, heavier, as you feel more and more at ease *(pause)*, your shoulders now *(pause)*, relaxed *(pause)*, more and more relaxed as a sense of heaviness replaces the sense of tension *(pause)*. Now your forehead and scalp *(pause)*. More relaxed, more at ease, your eyes *(pause)*, your lips *(pause)*, your tongue *(pause)*, your jaw *(pause)*, your throat now more and more relaxed *(long pause)*. Your neck is more relaxed, your chest is more and more relaxed. Now your upper back *(pause)*, your stomach and abdomen *(pause)*, letting the tension disappear. Your lower back *(pause)* and buttocks are more relaxed. Now with your legs *(pause)*, your thighs *(pause)*, and your calves, let the relaxation spread. Just allow any tension to drain away from *(pause)* your thighs *(pause)* and your calves. Allow your feet *(pause)* and now your toes and arches to become more and more relaxed *(pause)*, more and more relaxed.

Following the relaxation instructions, the group members are again asked to think of a number on the SUD scale that would describe their current level of relaxation or comfort. The group members are then told to count backward to themselves, slowly, from three to one and to open their eyes when they are ready. Post-relaxation-training SUD levels are then recorded. Group members are reassured that the absence of any decrement in SUD level or, perhaps, even an increase need not be a cause for concern. In some instances, the member may (1) be trying too hard to relax, (2) have ignored the caution not to overexert himself while tensing or (3) be preoccupied by distracting cognitions. There are many possible reasons for a small or negative change, but unless volunteered, the reason should not be pried out of the patient.

Next, the Relaxation Sequence (Appendix 12) with cues is handed out to assist the members' recall of the exercise during practice sessions.

Homework Assignment

The homework assignment is explained and the homework Assignment sheet for Session 2 is handed out with the Relaxation Practice Log (Appendix 8). (1) Group members are asked to continue practicing the BRR once daily for five minutes each session and to record the BRR practice session in their relaxation log. (2) Members are to practice the DMR once daily for 15 to 20 minutes and to record their progress in the relevant sections of the relaxation log. Practice sessions should be scheduled at times conducive for relaxation (for example, just prior to or following sleep can lead to falling asleep and not realizing the end point of relaxation). (3) Members are asked to read Part II of *Feeling Good* (pages 51–204) and (4) to contact their buddy. (5) Last, participants are asked to bring in a list of five or more situations in which they become anxious and/or depressed.

Feedback to Therapists

Feedback, both positive and negative, is solicited from the participants to aid the therapists in planning future sessions and to reinforce what has been learned during this session.

Personal Reminder Form

As in Session 1, Personal Reminder Forms are distributed to the group members. A copy is given to the group leader.

HOMEWORK ASSIGNMENT—SESSION 2

1. Practice BRR once daily for five minutes and make the appropriate notations on the relaxation log.
2. Practice DMR once daily for 15 to 20 minutes and make the appropriate notation on the relaxation log.
3. Read Part II of *Feeling Good*.
4. Contact buddy once during the week.
5. Make a list of situations during the week (or in the past) in which you found yourself to be inappropriately anxious, depressed, angry, guilty, or feeling any other extremely negative emotion.

THE COGNITIVE RESTRUCTURING
MODULE – SESSION 3

OVERVIEW

Attendance Taking, Homework Review, and Completion of A/P Sheets
Answering Questions on Homework Assignments
Collection of Relaxation Log, A/P Sheet, and Other Written Homework
New Material for Relaxation
Introduction to Cognitive Restructuring Theory
Discussion of Concept of Automatic Thoughts (ATs)
Personal Example of Leader Illustrating ATs
Externalization-of-Voices Technique Used to Demonstrate the Generation of
    Rational Responses
Eliciting Automatic Thoughts from Group Members regarding Group
    Treatment
Homework Assignment
Feedback from Group Members on This Session
Personal Reminder Form

Materials Needed:
    1. Attendance/Performance records (A/P) (Appendix 6)
    2. Relaxation Practice Log (Appendix 8)
    3. Blank NCR paper
    4. Homework Assignment sheet
    5. Personal Reminder Form (Appendix 10)

INTRODUCTION TO THE COGNITIVE RESTRUCTURING MODULE

Sessions 3, 4, 5, and 6 will be devoted in large part to skill training in the area of cognitive restructuring. This technique will be taught using the basic tenets of Aaron T. Beck and Albert Ellis, two major cognitive theorists. Beck's cognitive behavior therapy and Ellis's rational emotive therapy will be integrated in this module to instruct the participants in controlling their feelings by recognizing and challenging faulty thinking habits. The therapists present paradigms and personal examples to this end as well as assigning readings and written homework. In-group exercises include the role playing of distorted thoughts and their rational counterparts, with the group members gradually taking on more and more of a therapeutic role for each other. The therapists have as their goal for this module that each participant be able to demonstrate an understanding of cognitive restructuring and be able to apply it in at least mildly to moderately upsetting situations.

INTRODUCTION TO SESSION 3

Session 3 introduces the theory of cognitive restructuring. Briefly stated, this posits that inappropriately negative mood states are not produced by external circumstances but rather by the toughts or attitudes that one holds regarding these circumstances. Participants become acquainted with the concept of automatic thoughts or irrational cognitions, which can lead to dysfunctional moods such as extreme anger, sadness, guilt, and so on. The group leaders demonstrate how they themselves use the technique to identify and counter their own negative self-statements. Following this, automatic negative thoughts regarding being in a group are elicited from the group members, and the therapists demonstrate rational alternatives to this thinking through the use of role-playing and reverse role-playing techniques.

The homework assignment for this session includes continued reading in the area of cognitive restructuring as well as relaxation practice, buddy contact, and the recording of automatic thoughts identified during the coming week.

SESSION 3

Attendance Taking, Homework Review, and Completion of A/P Sheets

The administrative tasks are performed as in previous sessions. The homework assigned at the previous session included (1) daily practice of BRR with Relaxation Practice Log notations; (2) practice of DMR once daily as taught in previous session, tensing all muscle groups, and completion of Relaxation Practice Log; (3) read Part II of *Feeling Good*; (4) list five or more situations in the past week or in your past experience in which you became anxious and/or depressed; (5) contact buddy. Group members are reminded of the aforementioned assignments and are asked to make the appropriate notations on their A/P sheets as to compliance or noncompliance.

Answering Questions on Homework Assignments

Group members are encouraged to ask any questions they may have about the relaxation practice, the readings, or the collection of situations in which they become anxious or depressed. Patients commonly ask questions this session about problems in scheduling relaxation practice and in tensing muscles too strongly. The following is a list of typical problems and recommendations suggested by the group leaders:

Problem: Falling asleep during practice sessions at home.
Recommendation: The leaders regularly caution against practicing while in bed or in a reclining position. They also advise the participants to avoid practicing immediately before retiring or upon awakening. Falling asleep is not consistent with a practice schedule emphasizing the learning of a new skill, as it prevents the patient from experiencing the end state of increased relaxation. Consequently, if the patient wishes to use this technique for sleep induction, additional scheduled practice sessions are suggested.

Problem: Difficulty finding the time to practice.
Recommendation: Patients often explain that one reason for their need to attend the sessions has been their frenetic life-style. Consequently, they complain that to ask them to add relaxation practice sessions to their already overcommitted schedules is counterproductive and exacerbates their presenting problem. The group

leaders can respond to this objection by leading a discussion encouraging other group members to share the ways in which they have been able to make suggestions for finding convenient times and places for practice sessions (e.g., sitting on the bus or subway while commuting to and from work, closing the office door during lunchtime, or even practicing in the washroom).

Problem: Muscular pain during or following DMR practice sessions.

Recommendation: Patients not infrequently confuse the concept of working hard to learn the new relaxation skill with the amount of calories burned while practicing this new skill. They are reminded that some bodily states are only achieved with reduced effort (e.g., sleep, sexual arousal) and that the relaxed state is best attained by only slight tensing—not dramatic exertion.

Problem: The therapist's voice is believed to be integral to successful relaxation.

Recommendation: Patients are reassured that with sufficient practice they will become experts in their individual responses to relaxation and the soothing tones of the therapist's voice will be unnecessary to achieve high levels of relaxation.

Collection of Relaxation Log, A/P Sheet, and Other Written Homework

New Material for Relaxation

Pairing Scenes with DMR

Following the question-and-answer period, the group is introduced to an important adjunct to the DMR procedure. They will be asked to pair imagined scenes with the fully relaxed state achieved at the conclusion of the DMR practice session. This process of consistent association of the end point of the relaxation practice with the scenes is likened to a self-conditioning procedure. This conditioning of the mental image with the bodily state is designed to assist the patient in achieving a rapid and heightened state of relaxation. The intent is to empower these scenes, once brought to mind, with an ability to call up the state of physical relaxation, just as if the patient had gone through the full DMR procedure. Or, short of replacing the DMR procedure, the scenes imaged during DMR practice would speed up the relaxation process and enhance the end point.

Two types of scenes are introduced. Each scene is imaged utilizing as many sensory modalities as possible (namely, sight, sound, movement, touch, and smell). The process emphasizes actively experiencing the scene as real, not passively observing a picture in the mind. The first scene that is introduced, the pleasant scene, is often associated with nature, and the absence of other people; it is characteristically used in a calming mode to assist in slowing the body down (e.g., for sleep or sexual activity). Though each participant is free to choose his own, the following is used in the session as both an illustration and as a potential choice for a personal pleasant scene. Before the scene is presented, the leader names body parts in the order used in the prior DMR training exercise (Session 2). But the participants are instructed not to move their muscles, only to allow them to relax as in the latter part of that instructional set (pp. 59–60). The pleasant scene description follows:

> Now, I want you to imagine that you are lying on a beach, your eyes lightly closed, you are in your bathing suit, the bright sun is above you and you can see a bit of the sun sparkling through your lightly closed eyelids (long pause). You will also notice that you can see a ball, the bright orange ball of the sun. It feels as though it were lightly imprinted on top of your eyes, like a photographic negative. The warmth of the sand feels as though it were lightly baking your back as you lie there with the sun directly on top of you, making you feel very warm, lazy, and heavy. You can smell the salty sea and feel a soft breeze against your skin. Off in the distance you can hear a seagull or two and can hear the sounds of the waves come to the shore (long pause). Feel the warmth and the heaviness of your body (long pause). Just allow yourself to experience that now. With all your senses, make it very real for yourself, feel very, very relaxed. This is not a photograph; make it a real experience. Just try and make the scene all the more real to you (two-minute pause). And when you are ready you can just open your eyes, feeling comfortably refreshed, relaxed even more (pause) as you open your eyes, you will feel alert, comfortably refreshed and relaxed.

Following the presentation of the pleasurable scene and the two minutes of practice, the group members are given the opportunity briefly to discuss their experiences and the uses of the scene.

The second type of scene, the mastery or competency scene, is now introduced. It involves past or fantasized experiences associated with experiences of success or accomplishment. The event that is called to mind need not be momentous; it can be extremely mundane. The intent is to recapture or create a sense of control and well-being.

No scene is presented to the group, but, with their eyes lightly closed, they are instructed as follows:

> Please call to mind, as vividly as possible using all available senses and in an active mode, a scene in which you are feeling confident and in control.

This should be a scene where you have just accomplished something—it need not be of great moment. It may be that you have just put in the last piece of a 1,000-piece jigsaw puzzle, filled in the last word in the weekly crossword puzzle, just made your best soufflé, or just "kissed goodnight" on a date for the first time. Remember to use all your senses, to feel yourself in this past or fantasized scene *(two-minute pause).* And when you are ready, you can just open your eyes feeling comfortably refreshed, relaxed, and with a sense of competence and control. As you open your eyes, you will feel alert, comfortably refreshed, and relaxed.

The competency/mastery scene is most commonly used in situations where the patient is feeling tense because of some performance anxiety (e.g., making a speech). The intent is not so much to bring about a sense of absolute calm as to instill a sense of well-being and control.

The participants are asked to decide on one scene for each of the two categories and to imagine them for two minutes each following each DMR practice session. The patient is encouraged, when these relaxation skills are put into use, to employ the scenes as enhancers.

Introduction of Cognitive Restructuring Theory

Group members are next asked to share their second assignment, which was to make a list of situations during the week in which they had become anxious or depressed. A few of these situations are presented briefly by each member (see Table 3 for examples). This exercise serves as a lead-in to the following presentation of cognitive restructuring techniques.

TABLE 3. Examples of Situations Brought in by Group Members as Part of Their Homework

Assignment from Week 2

1. Driving to work every day past my estranged husband's apartment (where he is living with another woman)
2. Being caught in traffic and late for work
3. Being asked to do someone else's work in addition to my own
4. Coming home from work and finding that the house is a mess and no one has started dinner
5. Waiting up at night for my philandering husband to come home
6. Being given a writing assignment on a subject I know little about
7. Opening up my closet every morning and seeing that all my clothes are out of style
8. My mother calling to complain that I never call or write

The following introduction to cognitive restructuring (Beck, 1967; Ellis, 1962) is given to the group members by the co-therapists. This introduction is suggested as a model in that it purposely avoids technical language (jargon) so as to facilitate group members' understanding of the initial explanations.

Cognitive restructuring or Cognitive Behavior Therapy (CBT) is a self-help technique that can be used by virtually all of you to lessen or eliminate undesirable emotional reactions. The theory upon which CBT is based is that it is not situations or events which cause our extreme states of depression, anxiety, anger, or jealousy but the thoughts that we have about these events. Therefore, by changing our thoughts or attitudes, we can change our emotions. The first step is to catch yourself while you are thinking these thoughts. For example, when you are experiencing an unpleasant emotion that seems inappropriately severe, you stop and ask yourself "What am I saying to myself?" Once you've discovered a negative thought (e.g., a pessimistic statement about yourself, the future, or life in general), the next step is to ask yourself a question about that thought (e.g., "Am I certain about this?" or "Is there another possible explanation?" etc.). Your objective answers to these and other challenging questions are frequently more reasonable than your initial self-statements and will very likely result in a more moderate, more pleasant state of mind, including a reduction in emotional distress.

There is no claim that this technique will be a cure-all experience. Indeed, there will be occasions when you will suffer disappointments and losses and be treated shabbily. However, by employing a cognitive restructuring model, you will be able to assume greater control of your responses to these unpleasant events. Hence, with a less extreme reaction, you are likely to be able to respond more thoughtfully and with a greater measure of control. You also will be more likely to achieve your desired ends rather than to respond impulsively and "without thinking." Although the technique does not totally eliminate anxiety and depression from one's life, the extremity of these emotional states can be lessened through appropriate use of cognitive restructuring techniques. This group experience will provide you with a skill that you can use or not as you wish. For example, there are times when you might choose to remain sad, seemingly enjoying the extreme emotional state of depression. You might choose to remain in this negative feeling state despite having confidence that with some effort, cognitive restructuring techniques could lessen the distress.

The concepts of CBT should not be confused with "power of positive thinking" philosophies. CBT is not merely exchanging a positive thought for a negative one but rather recognizing and examining assumptions that lead to dysfunctional emotional states and then questioning and challenging these assumptions. The desired goal is not to transform a pessimistic thought to an optimistic one but rather to replace an automatic and unfounded irrational belief with one that is more objectively reasonable. These reasonable or rational thoughts are likely to lead to more functional and more appropriate emotional states.

Teaching Cognitive Restructuring Skills

Group members are reminded of the situations they have listed during the week in which they became anxious and/or depressed. The basic premise of CBT is then reemphasized—that is, it is not external situations which cause extreme negative emotions but rather what one says to himself about these situations.

The examples presented by the group members are mentioned as illustrations of negative emotions stemming from negative thinking. Any spontaneous reference by participants to negative thoughts is reinforced and used to lead into an explanation of automatic thoughts.

Discussion of Concept of Automatic Thoughts (ATs)

Group participants are reminded of the concept of ATs from their reading assignments in *Feeling Good*. ATs are described as thoughts that seem to appear immediately and habitually in certain situations. (Although any thoughts can be "automatic," for the purposes of CBT and this manual we will use the term *automatic thoughts* to represent negative, illogical thoughts about oneself, others, the world, or the future.) These thoughts often result in inappropriate and unnecessarily negative reactions. They appear to be part of one's repertoire and are triggered by different situations for different people. Patients often ask where these thoughts come from. The response is that they are learned earlier in life from (1) how we are treated by others, (2) how our role models feel about themselves and what they say to themselves, (3) what has been said to us about ourselves, and (4) our general life experiences. Beck *et al.* (1979) speak of the "cognitive triad"—that category of thinking, so typical of the depressive's cognitive style, which results in distorted and pessimistic views of the world, the future, and oneself.

To illustrate more clearly what an AT is, one of the group leaders will give a personal example of ATs in a particular situation.

Personal Example of Leader Illustrating ATs

In order to illustrate the concept of ATs and how these cognitions may result in inappropriate emotional states, one of the therapists gives an example from his own life. The problem situation and its accompanying automatic thoughts is first described in narrative form by the therapist. The automatic thoughts are then separated out for emphasis. The therapist presents his example at the outset for several reasons. The first is to establish the premise that everyone, regardless of his professional training, is prone to irrational lapses. This aids in alleviating the patients' tendency to label themselves as stupid or inferior for having these thoughts. The second reason is to model self-disclosure for the group members. Patients are often reluctant to speak in detail about personal problems in the group. They are frequently afraid of sounding ridiculous or of being the only ones who have ever felt this way. A third reason for the therapists to use personal examples is that their examples are often more interesting, more meaningful, and more realistic than the textbook or "canned" examples that could be used.

A sample therapist's example follows:

> The morning before leaving for a business trip, I found myself experiencing feelings of anxiety and unhappiness. These feelings were accompanied by gradually rising body tension (most noticeably stomach pains) and by a lack of energy. These symptoms were disconcerting, especially because there was much work to be done that day. Using the CBT technique, I asked myself, "What was I saying to myself?" That is, "What are my automatic thoughts?" I was able to uncover the following negative cognitions: (1) My desk is piled so high that I'll never see the top of it again. (2) Because my desk is so cluttered, I'll overlook something very important that I absolutely have to do before I leave. (3) I'll remember what I've forgotten while on the trip and it will ruin the trip for me. (4) The responsibilities that I will be neglecting will cause my colleagues problems; they will be angry with me and that will be awful. (5) I've taken on too many responsibiltiies and things will now fall apart while I'm gone.

Externalization-of-Voices Technique Used to Demonstrate the Generation of Rational Responses

The externalization-of-voices technique (Burns, 1980a), or role playing/reverse role playing (Beck *et al.*, 1979), is an exercise in which one person gives voice to or portrays negative automatic thoughts while the other counters those thoughts with more rational, objective responses. One can arrive at these more reasonable retorts by asking oneself "How would an objective observer view this situation?" "What is my evidence that my thought is the only interpretation of the situation?" "What could be an alternative explanation?"

To demonstrate this technique, one therapist role-plays his automatic thoughts from his personal problem situation while the other role-plays rational responses (RRs) to these thoughts. The specific directions for this role play include the following:

1. The person role-playing the negative automatic thoughts uses the pronoun *you* (e.g., "You'll never see the top of your desk again").

2. The person role-playing the more rational, reasonable, or objective voice uses the pronoun *I* (e.g., "My desk has looked like this before and I have managed to organize it and make order out of what seems to be chaos").

Illustrative responses to the remainder of the automatic thoughts can include the following:

AT: Because your desk is so cluttered you'll overlook something very important that you absolutely have to do.

RR: I still have time to look through the paperwork on my desk, make a list of my priorities, and do what I think is most important.

AT: You'll remember something you've forgotten while en route and it will ruin your trip.

RR: My list of priorities should help me remember the important things. If I do forget something, it won't be a catastrophe and I can choose not to worry about it on the trip.

AT: You will neglect some of your responsibilities, which will infuriate your colleagues and that will be awful.

RR: No one is perfect. If I do forget or neglect something, my colleagues may be temporarily irritated, but that doesn't mean they'd stay angry forever. Others do not have to think well of me at all times.

AT: You've assumed too many responsibilities and so things will fall apart while you're gone.

RR: As yet I have no evidence that I can't handle what I've undertaken. It is extremely unlikely that everything will fall apart while I'm gone. I can delegate anything that is crucial and that can't be completed before I leave.

The role play illustrated above is designed to model a way in which the group members can practice generating alternatives and more reasonable responses to their own set of dysfunctional thoughts. The responses generated need not be believed by the participants at this junction. The first step is merely being able to conjure up any possible alternatives to pessimistic predictions and other illogical assumptions. The use of the pronoun *you* by the voice role-playing the negative thoughts has two purposes. First, it is easier to recognize distortions when they are applied to someone other than oneself. Using the word *you* (e.g., "You never do anything right!") allows the owner of the statement a more objective view of this overgeneralization. Second, the use of *you* as an accusation makes it easier for one role-playing the rational voice to defend himself and to attack the illogic when the thoughts have been ostensibly disowned by their owner. While the dismissal of the irrational ATs is fostered, the owning of the rational responses is encouraged by the use of the pronoun *I* (e.g., "I obviously do some things right. I have many accomplishments I can point to"). The use of *I* is intended to promote identification with a more reasonable mode of thinking and to aid the speaker in internalizing a more functional set of attitudes.

The complete externalization of voice technique actually calls for role reversals. In this step the speaker in the irrational voice, after exhausting his automatic thoughts, is asked to speak in the rational voice and reply to his own ATs as well as any others generated by the opposing voice or other group members. The full technique is not used in this first exposure to cognitive restructuring, but it is used in Session 6, the last in this four-session module.

Eliciting Automatic Thoughts from Group Members regarding Group Treatment

Group members are now given the opportunity to generate their own automatic thoughts. They are asked to volunteer any negative reactions or predictions about being in group treatment. To make self-disclosure more comfortable, the directions to the group members can be as follows:

> Think about your initial and subsequent reactions to being in this group. For now, please focus on any negative thoughts you may have or have had in regard to yourself, other group members, and the progress you expect to make. If you are having difficulty generating any negative self-statements, you can generate ATs that anyone embarking on group treatment might experience.

The suggestion that one can attribute these thoughts to others usually suffices to break down any barriers to sharing dysfunctional thoughts.

The therapists make a list of all the appropriate thoughts that have been contributed. Questions are changed into statements and the therapists aid the participants in translating statements of feeling or fact into their irrational counterparts. At this stage, group members often have difficulty arriving at "pure" automatic thoughts, and it will be up to the therapists to gently transform their contributions in an instructive manner.

Some may regard the eliciting of ATs about membership in a group as courting trouble. We, on the contrary, have found this to be a most helpful exercise in building rapport with the group and in not side-stepping criticisms, be they justified or unjustified. It also provides the unique opportunity to have a forum in which to respond to their objections and to enlist the aid of objectors and observers alike in rebutting these criticisms.

The choice of this topic is also very convenient in that it is a common denominator. That is, every group member has group membership in common with every other.

Sample ATs from "Being in a Group" Exercise

1. "I won't be able to talk in front of all these people."
2. "My problems are worse than everyone else's."
3. "If I speak up, I'll sound stupid."
4. "I need the personal attention of individual therapy to get better."
5. "If the other group members find out what I'm really like, they won't like me."

The ATs generated by the group members will probably be variations of the examples given above. The leaders can now use these ATs in an externalization-of-voices role play, as was done for the therapist's personal example.

One therapist can role-play the ATs using the *you* voice (e.g., "You'll never be able to talk in front of all those people"). The other therapist can respond with a more logical counter thought such as "It's unlikely that I won't be able to speak in this group. Actually this is a safe situation in which to take risks. I may actually be more talkative here than in most group situations. Even if I'm not the most talkative person here, I can see that there is going to be much to learn and I can benefit a lot by listening, as well."

After role-playing several examples in a dialogue between the two therapists, the group members can begin taking turns and role-playing the ATs they've contributed using the *you* voice. The therapists will continue to role-play the rational responses using the *I* voice and will encourage the group members to do so as well. The following are possible counterresponses to the remaining ATs.

Sample Rational Responses to ATs from "Being in a Group" Exercise

AT: Your problems are worse than everyone else's.
RR: I can't know this early and maybe I never will know how severe other people's problems are in the group. Also, the difficulty of someone's problem is such a relative thing. Even if my problems are more difficult to solve, it doesn't mean that I can't do well for myself here.
AT: If you speak up, you'll sound stupid.
RR: I have no reason to believe that I sound stupid and much evidence that I won't. I'm also not here to win any intelligence contests. I'm here to learn and I can do that best by participating.

AT: You can't get what you need from a group. You need the personal attention of individual therapy to get better.

RR: I've already reaped some of the benefits of group therapy by recognizing that others have similar problems to my own. I've also seen that my goals coincide with the skills that will be taught in the group. It's just as likely that I'll gain as much or more from this experience as from individual treatment because I can learn from others as well as be motivated by their successes.

AT: If the other group members find out what you're really like, they won't like you.

RR: I don't know whether or not everyone would like me if they knew me well. Everyone doesn't need to like me for me to be happy. If there are some parts of me that I'd like to change, I can work on them. I don't have to show all to everyone, but this group is a safe place to find out how others react to me. It's a good opportunity to practice being myself and to *see* how others react to me.

Observing the role playing being used to deal with the group members' ATs about being in a group is one step closer to having them use the technique on themselves to counter their own, more personal illogical thinking. It is also a successive approximation of self-disclosure. Finally, it gives the therapists and other group members the opportunity to counter patients' misgivings about the group, which could impede their progress.

The next step will be to have the group members begin to identify their own ATs during the week between this session and next.

Homework Assignment

Homework Assignment sheets are handed out at this point. They contain the following:

1. Read Part III of *Feeling Good.*
2. Practice BRR once daily.
3. Practice DMR once daily, using both scenes.
4. Record 5 to 10 ATs during the week that resulted in unpleasant emotions. (Use the NCR paper provided.)
5. Speak with buddy once during the week.

Feedback from Group Members on This Session

As in former sessions, group members are asked to talk about what they found helpful in the session and to offer suggestions for changes in future sessions.

Personal Reminder Form

As at the end of each session, the Personal Reminder Forms are handed out. Group members are asked to complete them before they leave the group and to give the therapist one of the NCR copies.

HOMEWORK ASSIGNMENT—SESSION 3

1. Practice Benson's Relaxation Response (BRR) once daily for five minutes.
2. Practice Deep Muscle Relaxation (DMR) once daily, using both scenes.
3. Read Part III of *Feeling Good.*
4. Record 5 to 10 ATs during the week that resulted in unpleasant emotion. (Use the NCR paper provided.)
5. Make one buddy contact.

5

ENHANCING COGNITIVE
RESTRUCTURING SKILLS – SESSION 4

OVERVIEW

Attendance Taking, Homework Review, and Completion of A/P Sheets
Answering Questions on Homework Assignments
Collection of Relaxation Log, A/P Sheet, and Any Other Assignments Not
   Needed Later in the Session
New Material on Relaxation—Elimination of Tensing
Categorizing ATs Using Homework ATs and List of Cognitive Distortions
Introduction of Ellis's ABCDE Paradigm for Cognitive Restructuring
Group Practice of Cognitive Restructuring Skills
Homework Assignments
Feedback to Therapists
Personal Reminder Form

Materials Needed:
    1. A/P sheet (Appendix 6)
    2. Relaxation Practice Log (Appendix 8)
    3. Cognitive Distortions (Appendix 13)
    4. ABCDE paradigm (Figures 1, 2, and 3)
    5. Dispute Handles (Appendix 14)
    6. Homework Sheet for Cognitive Restructuring (Appendix 15)
    7. Homework Assignment sheet
    8. Personal Reminder Form (Appendix 10)

INTRODUCTION TO SESSION 4

In Session 4, participants learn to categorize their ATs according to a system developed by Beck (1979) and adapted by Burns (1980b). They are then exposed to Ellis's (1962) "ABCDE Paradigm for Cognitive Restructuring." Again, one leader uses a personal example to illustrate the use of the technique. The presentations and demonstrations serve to teach another, more structured version of cognitive restructuring which may appeal more to certain group members. For others it should reinforce what they've already learned about cognitive therapy from their reading and from the last session's presentation.

Categorizing the ATs aids patients in learning their own particular pattern of cognitive distortions (see Appendix 13). Group members can eventually learn to predict their own faulty logic by becoming familiar with their own distorted cognitive style. One goal is eventually to have them be able to practice in advance curative counterthoughts to their future cognitive errors.

SESSION 4

Attendance Taking, Homework Review, and Completion of A/P Sheets

The administrative tasks are performed as in previous sessions.

The homework assigned for session four included (1) reading Part III of *Feeling Good*; (2) once-daily practice of BRR, (3) once-daily practice of DMR with scenes; (4) record 5 to 10 automatic thoughts through the course of the week; and (5) make buddy contact. Group members are reminded of the aforementioned assignments and make appropriate notations on their A/P sheets as to compliance or noncompliance.

Answering Questions on Homework Assignments

The group members are encouraged to ask questions they may have about the new material from the previous week's session or from prior weeks. This includes the relaxation, reading, or CBT material.

Questions commonly arising at this point in the relaxation sequence are about the last session's new material (i.e., the relaxation-enhancing scenes). The following is a list of typical problems, recommendations suggested by the group leaders, and case examples for illustration:

Problem: Difficulty with the vividness of competency or pleasant scenes.
Recommendation: One common area of difficulty is the involvement of all senses in the imagery. The vividness of the scene suffers and

distractability increases when all possible senses are not included. Hence, the group members are urged to use multiple sensory modalities in their imagings. While it is not necessary to utilize *all* senses in constructing a scene in imagination, relying on one dominant sense often proves insufficient.

Case Example

A female patient chose for her pleasant scene the image of herself listening to her favorite Beethoven symphony. The image that she created used only her auditory sense. She complained in the group that she found herself easily distracted while imaging her scene. In attempting to enhance the image so as to bring on an increased level of relaxation, the patient was encouraged to concentrate on the pleasant feelings from the fabric of the couch on which she was lying, the dim lighting in her living room, the warmth from the fireplace, and the rich smell of the burning embers. Utilizing this enhanced image, the patient was successful in achieving a greater level of relaxation.

Problem: The imaged scene chosen brings on tension.

Recommendation: Patients often complain that any competency or mastery scene is tinged with anxiety for them and cannot be used to heighten relaxation. It is suggested that the group member may be choosing scenes from situations which are already extremely anxiety-producing for him. Patients are encouraged to look for areas of competency or mastery in less emotionally charged areas of their lives or in areas they may consider of lower priority. Another problem area while using the imagery is the patients' choice of "contaminated" material. That is, the patient will inadvertently conjure up scenes that have negative associations, either past or present. Less intense scenes, even if they may be less easily imaged, are prescribed. Patients are also reminded that competency scenes are often most helpful before an anxiety-producing event, when complete relaxation is not always the goal. Rather, a calm yet very alert state may be desirable.

Case Example

A patient complained that whenever she pictured herself mastering a situation at work, she found herself becoming only more tense, picturing all that she wanted yet to accomplish. She was encouraged to think of other non-work-related areas of competency and arrived at a very satisfying scene depicting herself reaping the rewards of her vegetable garden.

Case Example

A young man who had strong positive feelings about family ties and tradition called to mind the annual Thanksgiving family meal of his childhood for his "pleasant" scene. Unfortunately, as he concentrated on details to enhance the scene, he found himself becoming increasingly agitated and consequently less relaxed. Only as he sought to recreate the scene in greater detail did he begin to remember the familial acrimony, unpleasant scenes, and underlying feuding of past years. By way of remediation, the patient was urged to use a more neutral scene even if it seemed less real or personal to him.

Problem: Any scene is distracting and does not enhance the relaxation process.

Recommendation: Occasionally, a patient will complain that virtually any scene is distracting. He is then given the option of using no scene at all or using a sensorily deprived scene, such as lying in bed in total darkness. Another, similarly neutral scene would be being covered with sand on a beach, emphasizing the sense of warmth and total envelopment.

Collection of Relaxation Log, A/P Sheet, and Any Other Assignments Not Needed Later in the Session

Relaxation logs and A/P sheets are collected at this point. Group members are asked to keep their lists of automatic thoughts until later in the session.

New Material on Relaxation — Elimination of Tensing

Reducing Tensing

The new relaxation element to be introduced in this session is the instruction to the patient to begin reducing the amount of tensing he does prior to relaxing each successive muscle group during DMR practice. In the original instruction for DMR, the patient is instructed to tense each muscle group sufficiently to notice a slight level of discomfort. The removal of this discomfort in the practice session served to underscore the positive feelings attendant on relaxation. The utility of this instructional technique diminishes over the following two weeks of practice. In fact, the results of DMR are enhanced by eliminating the preliminary tensing. This step is achieved through the *gradual* reduction of the prior tensing element in each successive practice session. The patient is told successively to drop out a bit of the prior tensing. By the end of the week intervening between group meetings, the patient is no longer tensing at all. The practice session will then resemble part 2 of the training session (see Session 2), where muscle groups are successively relaxed without any movement on the part of the relaxer.

Relaxation

At this point the therapist leads the group through part 2 of the entire relaxation sequence, allowing one minute for each of the two enhancing scenes.

Categorizing ATs Using Homework ATs and List of Cognitive Distortions

Homework assignment 4 from last session was to list 5 to 10 ATs generated in the course of the week. The intent was to raise the sensitivity of the members, to have them recognize that they are likely to generate these types of thoughts (i.e., distortions) in a variety of situations, and that an excellent clue to the presence of such thinking is the residue of negative feelings.

The leader then records a number (approximately 12 to 15) of ATs from the participants by requesting that volunteers call out an AT, which the leaders then write on a blackboard or on newsprint.

Following this exercise, a list of 10 cognitive distortions (Burns, 1980b) is distributed (see Appendix 13). This list is an expansion of Beck's (1976) classification of the types of dysfunctional thinking people are likely to engage in—particularly those prone to mood disorders. The leaders then call for the participants to categorize their own ATs that are listed on the board. For those types not listed, the leaders may use any from the leader's example given at last session or generated by the members in last session's exercise about "being in a group." The participants will be somewhat familiar with this list from their reading. The leaders then collect one copy of the homework assignment (list of 5 to 10 ATs) to review for degree of understanding of the AT concept.

The categorization of types of dysfunctional thinking is stressed in this phase of the module. The intent is to familiarize the group member with his particular style of distorting reality as he talks to himself about his perception of himself, the world, and the future. The classification system assists in the recognition of a personal mood-altering process of thinking and can facilitate the patient's task of changing this style of dysfunctional thinking.

An example of a personal style would be that of a man who, upon being rebuffed when asking a woman out for a date, would think:

"No one will ever go out with me." (Fortune-telling error, all-or-nothing thinking)

"Sally will tell all the gang about this and I'll be the laughing stock." (Fortune-telling error, catastrophizing)

By contrast, an identically unfortunate young man whom Joanne saw fit to turn down might think:

"It's not fair that Joanne would do this to me." ("Should" statement)

"I'm a failure." (Labeling)

Recognizing styles of distorted thinking is especially important when using Ellis's model (Ellis, 1962) for cognitive restructuring. Ellis employs specific strategies (disputes) that are more appropriate for some types of distortions than others. The following is a more structured approach to cognitive behavior therapy which was developed by Ellis. The less structured Beck approach was presented first to illustrate the end result of the cognitive restructuring process. The Ellis model breaks the process down into its various components and may be more attractive or more understandable to certain group members. The authors have found a combination of the two approaches to be more generally effective than either model alone.

Introduction to Ellis's ABCDE Paradigm for Cognitive Restructuring

As in the last session, the teaching of a model for cognitive restructuring is preceded by the presentation of a personal example by one of the group leaders. The personal example is initially presented in narrative form; following this, a formal presentation is made describing Ellis's paradigm for cognitive restructuring. The therapist's example is then broken down to conform to the paradigm.

An illustration of a therapist's personal example in narrative form follows:

I was in the midst of having a major construction job completed on my home when the contractor informed me that he'd be leaving the area immediately following completion of the contract. I was feeling anxious— at a loss for words—and abruptly ended the conversation with him.

I then began brooding about how unfair it was that he had not told me about this sooner and fearing that he would do a sloppy job in finishing the work, for which I would have no recourse.

After catching myself catastrophizing about these events, I asked myself several questions about my worries, like "After all, do I have a right to determine where my contractor will be living forever? Did he promise me he'd stay in the area? How do I know that he planned this all along or knew about it any sooner than he'd told me? How did I know for sure that he'd do a poor job of finishing and if he did, wouldn't there be some legal or financial recourse available to me?"

In answering these questions, I reminded myself that "Of course being the contractor's customer gives me no right over his future residence of future occupation. He made no promises to me in any case. Even if he had been deceiving me, he has done a very satisfactory job thus far. (Even his subcontractors have said so!) It's not unexpected that he would continue with this quality of workmanship. If he doesn't, I still would have the portion of his fee I'm holding as per our contract. I could continue to hold it until I'm satisfied with the job and until he has made suitable provisions for a warranty on his work."

Following this internal dialogue, I felt calmer. I called my contractor later that evening and was appropriately fluent and assertive. The provisions for warranty work seemed satisfactory and the good rapport we had established was continued.

Ellis's model for cognitive restructuring follows the easily remembered sequence of ABCDE, which describes both the process of dysfunctional thinking and a model for its remediation. The paradigm and detailed explanation follow (the amount of theoretical background may, of course, be tailored to the needs and interests of the participants):

A—Activating Event
B—Belief System
  iB—Irrational Belief
  rB—Rational Belief
C—Consequence
D—Dispute
E—Effect
  aE—Affective Effects
  bE—Behavioral Effects
  cE—Cognitive Effects

The *activating event* (A) is the situation (including daydreams or recollections) which is *initially* thought to cause the unpleasant or negative emotional states.

The *belief system* (B) is the mediating event (i.e., thoughts, cognitions)

$$A \nrightarrow C$$

$$A \;\rightarrow\; B \;\rightarrow\; C$$

FIGURE 1. A representation of the basic premise of the origin of emotions. The activating event (A) does not lead directly to the consequence (C); the belief system (B) mediates.

linking the activating event and the consequence. *Irrational beliefs* (iB; previously called ATs) are those cognitions which tend to lead to extreme negative emotional or physical states. *Rational beliefs* (rB; previously called RRs) are those cognitions which replace the irrational beliefs as a result of the successful completion of the cognitive restructuring exercise. They tend to be less extreme in content and result in a reduction in the extremity of the previously experienced negative emotional or physical state.

The *consequence* (C) is the emotional state commonly viewed as being caused by the activating event but which actually results from the intervening variable, the belief system (see Figure 1). Typical consequences include extreme negative emotional states (e.g., excessive anger, jealousy, guilt, depression or anxiety) or physical states (e.g., muscular tension and gastrointestinal distress).

The *dispute* (D) is used in the process of challenging the logic or reasonableness of the irrational belief system. Group members are taught to question the authenticity of the belief system that gives rise to discomforting consequences. They are taught a format for calling into question the logical foundations of their irrational beliefs. This format begins with stock "dispute handles" (see Appendix 14). With sufficient practice, the disputes are made more specific to the situation with reduced reliance on these "handles."

A dispute is formulated for each of the irrational beliefs encountered in a troubling situation. The responses to the disputes become the rational beliefs that supplant or are substituted for the irrational beliefs,

$$A + iB \rightarrow C$$

$$A + rB \rightarrow \begin{cases} aE \;(\text{Affective}) \\ bE \;(\text{Behavioral}) \\ cE \;(\text{Cognitive}) \end{cases}$$

FIGURE 2. A diagram of the cognitive model of mood disorders. The activating event (A) leads to undesirable consequences (C) or desirable effects (E) depending upon the irrational (iB) or rational (rB) belief system employed.

hence denying what had seemed to be the automatic linking of the consequences to the activating event.

Subscribing to the new rational beliefs results in more positive affective (aE), behavioral (bE), and cognitive (cE) effects (see Figure 2). Affective changes might, for example, include mood elevation and a reduction in anger. Behavior changes are likely to lead to an increase in available goal-directed energy and the accomplishment of tasks previously inhibited by focusing one's attention on the problem as opposed to the solution. Cognitive changes are likely to lead to positive changes in attitude which may be generalized to many other situations (see Figure 3).

At the outset, the patient's strict adherence to the paradigm is recommended. No mention is made of shortcuts in using the technique, though the therapists might acknowledge that a paper-and-pencil analysis is not always necessary. In a later session (Session 5), a modification of this paradigm is introduced which does not use disputes as a means of arriving at rational beliefs. This latter format is employed in the Advanced Homework Sheet (see Appendix 16). Experience has shown that cognitive restructuring is best learned first through the ABCDE par-

A
Being fired from the job

iB
"I'll never find another job."

D
"Do I know for certain?"

rB
"I'm certainly not pleased that I
lost my job, but I don't know what
the future will bring. My next
position may be just as likely to be
better as it is to be worse."

C
Anxiety, depression, and headaches

aE   Feeling less anxious and depressed and more hopeful about the future.
bE   "I began job hunting."
cE   "This is not the only good job I could have. Out of this crisis can come a welcome
     opportunity."

FIGURE 3. A diagram of the application of the cognitive model to a reactive depression.

adigm and a corresponding rigid adherence to its format. However, patients may rapidly grow tired of its numerous steps. Consequently, a more rapid analysis is later welcomed by the patient and encourages the continued practice that is so necessary in the patient's adaptation to a modified cognitive approach (see Session 5).

The first therapist reminds the group in summary form of his earlier personal example. The second therapist then proceeds to fit each part of the example into the ABCDE format (see Appendix 17).

The use of a blackboard or newsprint taped to the wall of the group room is important for more effective teaching of the model at this point. Only after the example has been presented in written form by the therapist is the handout (Appendix 17) distributed.

A list of Ellis's "Basic Irrational Ideas" (Ellis, 1962) is distributed next (Appendix 18). A therapist then demonstrates the similarity between the IB's in his personal example and Ellis's irrational beliefs.

Next, a list of "Dispute Handles" (Appendix 14) is distributed. The other therapist illustrates how the use of various disputes in the example corresponds to those listed in Appendix 14. Emphasis is placed on the dispute as a means of challenging the belief system linking the consequence to the activating event. By asking a critical question about this automatic linking, the logic of the consequence resulting from the activating event is put into question.

In many ways, especially when this is a beginning skill, the success of a CBT analysis depends very heavily on the dispute section. As was stated before, the dispute section of CBT analysis is often made optional, but we find it to be an important component of CBT when it is taught in a group composed of patients with a range of intelligence, verbal skills, and cognitive styles.

It is not uncommon for patients to object to the use of the word *rational* or in some ways to confuse the term *rational* with *rationalizing*. To illustrate the difference, "rationalizing" can be defined for the group members as the use of excuses or justifications to explain away anything that is undesirable. "Rational thinking," on the other hand, can be described as the result of objectively questioning the evidence at hand when experiencing extreme unproductive emotions and responding to those questions with more reasonable replies. Rational thinking reflects a more realistic, objective, and dispassionate appraisal of the environment. These more reasonable cognitions are likely then to result in a more comfortable and productive emotional state. Therefore, the term *reasonable* or *realistic* can be substituted for *rational*, and later the terms may be used in parallel so as to lessen the likelihood of the patient confusing *rational thinking* with *rationalizing*.

The use of the term *irrational idea* or *irrational belief* is also often objected to, especially when the patient is not thoroughly convinced of the irrationality of his underlying thoughts. This is especially the case when the patient is taking a leap of faith in simply entertaining the idea that his belief system is leading to self-defeating behaviors and negative emotional states. Problems attendant to the use of the term *irrational belief* are avoided by substituting (as we have) the term *automatic thought* (Beck, 1967). In addition, homework sheets are distributed which use both terms (Appendixes 15 and 16).

Other common objectives and worries of group members can be anticipated and responded to prophylactically. One typical worry of a group member first learning about a cognitive restructuring approach to negative emotions is that the technique is too difficult or cumbersome to be a practical way to get relief from personal discomfort. Group members are reassured that rational thinking is a skill that comes more easily with practice and that at times might even become more "automatic" than irrational thinking. They are told that at the outset, however, such thinking is difficult to learn. Like any new, complex skill (e.g., playing tennis, playing a musical instrument, driving a car), it requires time, patience, practice, and a willingness to appear or feel awkward when it is first attempted. Group members practice each component part of the technique and then put the separate components together as part of a group exercise before they are sent out on their own to complete a homework assignment. The exercise consists of giving the group an activating event that seems to reflect a common experience. For most of our groups, the area that most likely reflects a common experience is a job-related problem. However, for groups where the bulk of members are nonworking or non-career-oriented, themes of domestic chores, childrearing, or relationships with friends are easily substituted. These initial problem areas are surely not the only ones common to group members. They are, however, relatively "safe" issues requiring a lesser degree of risk taking and self-disclosure when discussed in the group. In later sessions the group is led into more personal areas of concern (e.g., intimate interpersonal relationships, self-doubts, and feelings of personal inadequacy).

Group Practice of Cognitive Restructuring Skills

One typical completed group exercise is found in Appendix 19. The group leaders provide the activating event, which requires relatively little risk-taking yet is nonetheless a likely common problem area. Once the activating event (A) is announced and a list of likely somatic, behavioral, and negative affective states (C) is generated, the group is asked to generate potential (though not necessarily their own) irrational beliefs (iBs) about this event. The group then arrives at disputes (D) to the irrational beliefs (iBs). The answers to these disputes become the rational beliefs (rBs). The exercise ends in hypothesizing likely affective (aEs), behavioral (bEs), and cognitive (cEs) effects.

The group is now presented with a completed example (as can be found in Appendix 19) in handout form as a model to follow during the week when filling out their own CBT analysis of a personal problem situation. Blank CBT homework sheets (Appendix 15) are also distributed. The group members are asked to complete two homework sheets for the following session. They are told to be prepared to discuss at least one of these sheets in the group. The other may be of a more personal nature which they can elect not to reveal to the group.

The decision to ask that two homework sheets be completed and the option not to share one of them is the first step toward self-disclosure as well as working out more personal problems in a CBT format. There are several potential benefits for the group member in writing out an example of a more personal nature. First, even though it need not be shared, he is engaging in an approximation of self-disclosing behaviors which is akin to self-disclosure in the group. Writing out an example is closely related to actually revealing it, as it entails formulating the language descriptive of the problem. Often, this approximation of disclosure (i.e., writing it down) and, it is hoped, making an effort to deal with it in a rational, solution-oriented manner sufficiently defuses its "horribleness" so that the patient finds himself willing, if not eager, to share the example with the group. The example provided (Appendix 20) illustrates the case of a patient who wrote out the CBT homework sheet solely for her own scrutiny, because of its intense personal nature. However, she followed this homework sheet with an exercise dealing with her reluctance to disclose her homework assignment to the group. This latter exercise (see Appendix 21) was so successful that she felt ready to disclose her more personal example at the next group meeting. Most people would readily acknowledge that a woman's thoughts during sexual intercourse with her spouse are among the more private of interpersonal events. Yet she reported that, through the use of CBT, she was able to share this homework example comfortably with the group.

While it is not suggested that all group members will be so readily open to share the most personal of life events, especially so early in the life of the group, a homework assignment with the option of nonpublic disclosure can be an effective catalyst for taking increasingly greater personal risks.

Homework Assignments

The assignment for next session includes (1) reading part IV of *Feeling Good,* (2) the completion of two CBT homework sheets (as explained above), (3) calling the assigned buddy, and (4) practicing the relaxation exercises with the appropriate notations on the Relaxation Practice Log.

Group members are reminded that they will be asked to share one of their CBT homework sheets with the other participants during the following session. This reminder appears to aid in compliance with the assignment as well as ensuring that the group member is not caught unawares or pressured into revealing personal issues before he feels prepared to do so.

Feedback to Therapists

As in previous sessions, at least five minutes is allotted for feedback to the therapists on the positive and negative reactions of group members to the session.

Personal Reminder Form

As in previous sessions, the participants are asked to fill out the Personal Reminder Forms (on NCR paper) that serve both as prompts for them in reinforcing the learning experience and as an additional source of feedback to the therapists.

HOMEWORK ASSIGNMENT—SESSION 4

1. Arrive at rational responses to 5 to 10 ATs from the past week's homework by using dispute handles on blank NCR paper.
2. Complete two CBT homework sheets (Appendix 15), with at least one to be shared with the group next session.
3. Read *Feeling Good,* Part IV.
4. Practice BRR once daily.
5. Practice DMR once daily, eliminating tensing.
6. Contact buddy.

ENHANCING COGNITIVE RESTRUCTURING SKILLS – SESSION 5

OVERVIEW

Attendance Taking, Homework Review, and Completion of A/P Sheets

Answering Questions on Homework Assignments

Collection of Relaxation Log, A/P Sheet, and Any Other Assignments Not Needed Later in the Session

New Material on Relaxation

Request Volunteers to Describe a Successfully Completed CBT Homework Sheet

Request Volunteer to Share a Problem That Could Be Worked on in the Group Using the CBT Model

Collection of Anonymous Situations with Corresponding ATs to Be Worked on in the Group (Optional)

Solicitation of Additional Volunteers to Work on Their Own Problems (Optional)

Introduce Advanced CBT Homework Sheet

Homework Assignment

Feedback from Group Members on This Session

Personal Reminder Form

Materials Needed:
1. A/P sheet (Appendix 6)
2. Relaxation Practice Log (Appendix 8)
3. Advanced Homework Sheet for Cognitive Restructuring (Appendix 16)
4. Homework Assignment Sheet
5. Personal Reminder Form
6. Identical sheets of paper and pens (optional)

INTRODUCTION TO SESSION 5

By Session 5 the group members have been exposed to two sessions of cognitive restructuring and many are likely to have had at least some success in countering dysfunctional thinking. Participants are encouraged to share their successes or partial successes with the technique. This sharing models for others how the technique can be used for a variety of problems and instills more confidence in the method for those still dubious about its utility.

After this positive beginning, the group members are invited to bring up problems they are having with this newly acquired skill. They can present homework with which they are having difficulty or a troubling situation for which they need some help, identifying and/or countering maladaptive thoughts.

This session lends itself more to group interaction and the sharing of personal issues than any of the preceding sessions. The advantages of teaching this skill in a group become apparent as group members begin to offer helpful, rational responses for each other in greater quantity and perhaps quality than could be generated by any one therapist.

SESSION 5

Attendance Taking, Homework Review, and Completion of A/P Sheets

The administrative tasks are performed as in previous sessions.

The homework assigned from Session 4 included (1) arrive at rational responses to the 5 to 10 ATs collected during the previous week, making use of the dispute handles (Appendix 14) on homework sheet; (2) read *Feeling Good*, Part IV; (3) practice BRR once per day; (4) practice DMR once per day; and (5) contact buddy.

Group members are reminded of the aforementioned assignments and make appropriate notations on their A/P sheets as to compliance or noncompliance.

Answering Questions on Homework Assignments

Group members are encouraged to ask questions they may have about the new material from last week's session or from prior sessions. This includes the relaxation training, readings, or CBT material.

Problems commonly encountered at this point in the relaxation sequence typically include questions about dropping out the tensing component of the procedure as well as concerns about not having "gotten it"—that is, not yet achieving the expected level of proficiency in the relaxation skill. The following is a list of problems, corresponding recommendations suggested by the group leaders, and case examples for illustration:

Problem: Parts of the body do not get relaxed without the prior tensing technique; when the tensing is dropped out, certain body parts will remain tense.

Recommendation: The prior tensing technique is originally taught to facilitate the recognition of the sensation of tension in various muscle groups. Upon the release of the tightened muscle, relaxation rebounds, thus enhancing the sensation of comfort and relaxation. This lends credibility to the DMR training process but does not necessarily result in a satisfactory state of overall relaxation. Clinical experience suggests that relaxation is enhanced through dropping out the prior tensing procedure. The patient can be encouraged to reduce the prior tensing more slowly for these particularly troubling body parts but to move toward the ultimate goal of doing no tensing and engaging in no movement at all to achieve the relaxed state.

Problem: The DMR is just not working the way it should.

Recommendation: DMR requires weeks of practice. The initial learning experience is a gradual one, and not necessarily consistently rewarding, especially if attempted in situations that would tax someone with even a highly developed skill. Three mistakes are commonly made: (a) attempting too early to use the technique in crisislike or overwhelming situations; (b) not recognizing a heightened level of tension early in the sequence, *before* feeling overwhelmed; and (c) not appreciating that this skill, like many others (swimming, driving), requires practice before it can be used to challenge formidable problems.

Case Example

A male patient had a heated argument with his boss. Upon returning to his office, he remembered his DMR training and attempted to use it, with negligible results. Upon recounting this "failure" to the group, he was reassured that this was a very demanding situation for the DMR technique and surely too demanding for the patient at this level of inexperience. Other stress-reducing techniques and more practice were indicated.

Collection of Relaxation Log, A/P Sheet, and Any Other Assignments Not Needed Later in the Session

Relaxation logs and A/P sheets are collected at this point. Group members are asked *not* to turn in their rational responses to their automatic thoughts at this time, as they will be used later in the session.

New Material on Relaxation

Differential Relaxation

The versatility of DMR is most apparent when teaching the concept of keeping one area or several areas of the body relaxed while others are appropriately tensed or in vigorous use. This is called differential relaxation. Participants learn that they need not frown when grasping a pencil or tighten their stomach muscles while driving a car. Different body parts can be specifically relaxed at different times (e.g., the beginnings of a tension headache can be eliminated by concentrating on relaxing the frontalis muscle alone).

Group members are then asked to relax a specific body area (e.g., the face) while maintaining the body posture they had assumed while listening to the brief didactic presentation, thus practicing the relaxation of one specific body area at a time.

Request Volunteers to Describe Successfully Completed CBT Homework Sheets

Group members are asked, in turn, to discuss how successful they felt in completing the new CBT homework sheet. Those who feel a greater sense of accomplishment are asked to share theirs first. It is important to deal with the more successful homework examples first in order to provide a model for others and also to establish the fact that the technique can be useful, even this early in the learning sequence. The volunteer is asked to label his cognitive distortions and also to include the dispute handles he used to arrive at the rational responses.

Request Volunteer to Share a Problem That Could Be Worked on in the Group Using the CBT Model

In this section the participants are requested to bring up ATs that they were unable to counter or even emotionally distressing situations in which they were unable to identify their ATs. The group can then work together in helping the volunteer to come up with more reasonable ways of thinking about the situation. This activity aids in fostering group cohesion, gives everyone practice in disputing cognitive distortions, and is the beginning of lessening dependence on the group leaders. Initially the leaders are more active, gradually decreasing their participation as the group members become more facile with the cognitive restructuring technique.

Collection of Anonymous Situations with Corresponding ATs to Be Worked on in the Group (Optional)

For various reasons group members are often reluctant to bring up personal situations to be dealt with in this group. If there are no or too few volunteers to present success experiences or problems, the group leaders can ask members to anonymously write down situations they found distressing and the accompanying ATs. Identical sheets of paper and pens are handed out to preserve anonymity. These ATs are collected and then selected one by one at random by the group members, who read them as though they were their own. This exercise is very similar to the second warm-up exercise in Session 1 (p. 43), the secrets game. The group joins the leaders in disputing the ATs and replacing them with more logical responses. The method of using anonymous ATs has the advantage of allowing the group members to hear alternative ways of thinking about their situations without having to self-disclose earlier than they feel prepared to. A disadvantage is that the group member presenting another's situation may not be able to "do it justice," and the owner of the problem may feel frustrated. Fortunately this reaction is often articulated upon questioning and the group itself asks to move on, having each present his or her own personal example.

Solicitation of Additional Volunteers to Work on Their Own Problems

If the group does decide that they are ready and willing to volunteer situations or thoughts for which they'd like the group's help and there is time remaining, additional problem areas can be addressed at this time.

Introduce Advanced CBT Homework Sheet

The Advanced Homework Sheet for Cognitive Restructuring (Appendix 16) is distributed and the group members' attention is directed toward how it differs from the original homework sheet (Appendix 15). The directions emphasize rating and rerating degrees of emotion experienced and degrees of belief in one's thoughts. In addition, the use of dispute handles is not included.

The rationale for adding the rating and rerating of the degree of unpleasant emotion experienced is that the patient can begin to see that he is making some headway in controlling his mood, if only by small increments. This can aid in countering the all-or-nothing thinking syndrome of "I tried it and I still feel blue, therefore it doesn't work."

Another advantage to rating and rerating one's thoughts is that one can also begin to see successive increases in the degree of belief in a rational counterthought and a corresponding decrease in one's commitment to the original automatic thought. This, too, can challenge a frequent complaint of newcomers to CBT which is "What good does it do me to write down these rational responses if I don't believe them anyway?" Requiring the learner to assign a number to how much he believes in an automatic thought or its rational counterpart can show gradual changes in the most firmly held dysfunctional cognitions.

The dispute section has not been included in the advanced homework sheet because it is seen as an aid that may no longer be needed by the patient except perhaps with particularly recalcitrant ATs. The homework sheets are designed as a steady progression toward eventually having the patient do most of his cognitive restructuring mentally, resorting to paper and pencil only in the most difficult situations.

Homework Assignment

Homework assignment sheets are now distributed; they contain the following directions:

1. Complete reading *Feeling Good* (the last chapter is optional).
2. Practice BRR once daily.
3. Practice DMR once daily, using differential relaxation.
4. Complete one advanced CBT homework sheet to share with the group (additional ones are optional).
5. Contact buddy.

Feedback from Group Members on This Session

As in past sessions, at least five minutes is allotted for feedback to the therapists on what the group members found to be helpful this session and what changes they would like to make in the future.

Personal Reminder Form

The Personal Reminder Forms are distributed and group members are asked to fill them out before leaving the group. The therapists collect one copy and the participants retain the other.

HOMEWORK ASSIGNMENT—SESSION 5

1. Complete reading *Feeling Good* (the last chapter is optional).
2. Practice BRR once daily.
3. Practice DMR once daily, employing the differential relaxation.
4. Complete one advanced CBT homework sheet to share with the group (additional sheets are optional).
5. Contact buddy.

ENHANCING COGNITIVE RESTRUCTURING SKILLS – SESSION 6

OVERVIEW

Attendance Taking, Homework Review, and Completion of A/P Sheets
Answering Questions on Homework Assignments
Collection of Relaxation Log and A/P Sheet, but Not Advanced CBT Homework Sheet
New Material on Relaxation
Solicitation of CBT Problems to Work on Using the Externalization-of-Voices Technique
Homework Assignment
Feedback to Therapists
Personal Reminder Form

Materials Needed:
  1. A/P sheet (Appendix 6)
  2. Relaxation Practice Log (Appendix 8)
  3. Blank NCR paper
  4. Homework assignment sheet
  5. Personal Reminder Form (Appendix 10)

INTRODUCTION TO SESSION 6

Session 6 is the last session to deal formally with the teaching of the cognitive restructuring skill. However, the technique will be used continually throughout the remainder of the group experience. For this session, success experiences with the homework may again be solicited, but the main emphasis is on drilling the participants in the use of the method. The therapists' major role is to elicit the automatic thoughts related to a particular group member's situation which engender a negative mood state. Following this, more and more responsibility is given to the participants to act as therapists for each other, thereby practicing eventually to become their own therapists in stressful situations.

During this session, the group leaders try to make sure that each member has enough understanding of the technique to be able to continue to refine it and eventually make it his own. All the participants may or may not feel that they are able to control their moods by the end of the group. The goal, however, is that by the end of this session the group members will be able to continue building their skill levels on their own.

SESSION 6

Attendance Taking, Homework Review, and Completion of A/P Sheets

The administrative tasks are performed as in previous sessions.

The homework assigned in the previous session included the following: (1) practice BRR once a day, (2) practice DMR once a day, (3) complete advanced CBT homework sheet, (4) complete *Feeling Good,* and (5) contact buddy.

Group members are reminded of the aforementioned assignments and make appropriate notations on their A/P sheets as to compliance or noncompliance.

Answering Questions on Homework Assignments

As in the past sessions, group members are encouraged to ask questions about any material previously covered. This includes the relaxation training, readings, and cognitive restructuring material.

Some problems covering the relaxation material and corresponding recommendations from the group leaders follow:

Problem: The patient falls asleep while practicing the DMR.
Recommendation: The patient who practices the DMR immediately
   before going to sleep, immediately upon awakening, or while in
   a reclining position may become sleepy or actually fall asleep. This
   can be avoided by choosing more appropriate times of day and by
   practicing in a more upright position.

Problem: It is difficult to find time to do the required number of practice sessions for the DMR (once or twice daily), BRR (once daily), and differential relaxation (daily).

Recommendation: Participants are encouraged to view the relaxation practice sessions as positive, life-enhancing events rather than minor (or major) irritants. (Some CBT might be in order here to look at the ATs surrounding "having to practice.") As the patient becomes increasingly adept at DMR, practice sessions should become more rewarding and actually require less time to complete. Group members can also be reminded that many who come to these groups have overscheduled themselves, and that they will be learning ways to prioritize their activities later in the group.

Problem: The patient encounters difficulty in setting the stage for relaxation and confusion as to how important quiet, freedom from interruptions (e.g., visitors, phone calls), and a comfortable chair actually are.

Recommendation: The great emphasis is upon frequent, regular practice. The setting is important and obvious interruptions and distractors can substantially inhibit the learning process. However, when choices must be made, practice under poor conditions is better than no practice at all. The patient is urged to find the best practice environment he can under his particular circumstances.

Collection of Relaxation Log and A/P Sheet, but Not Advanced CBT Homework Sheets

The advanced homework sheets are retained by the group members for discussion later in the session.

New Material on Relaxation

Each patient is likely to have specific parts of his body which will be more resistant to relaxation procedures. At this point participants are asked to describe these problems and discuss how to bring these problem areas into line. The basic approach is to counsel perserverence. Most troublesome areas will respond to the procedures already described in previous sessions. Often patients will become discouraged and be willing to tolerate an unnecessary level of tension in their bodies. Reassurance and urging can often bring the patient to be less tolerant of this level of discomfort.

Solicitation of CBT Problems to Work on Using the Externalization-of-Voices Technique

Group members are encouraged to discuss the advanced CBT homework sheets they have brought to share with the group. A volunteer or volunteers are requested to bring up difficulties they are having with the technique and/or problems they would like to deal with using the CBT method. The therapists can aid the volunteer in describing the situation or activating events, labeling the negative emotions, rating the degree of emotional distress, and listing the ATs. An explanation is again given regarding how to employ the externalization-of-voices technique (see Session 3), with the volunteer presenting his ATs in the second person (e.g., "You'll never get better."). The rest of the group and the therapists use the first person singular to rebut the ATs (e.g., "I'm learning new techniques and I'm making changes. I can't expect to turn around many years of habitual negative thinking in a few short weeks.").

Once the volunteer is beginning to appear somewhat convinced of the reasonableness of the rational counterthoughts or at least has run out of arguments (i.e., ATs), the roles should be reversed, allowing the volunteer an opportunity to espouse the rational arguments. This step is very important in determining the degree to which the patient has at least heard the more objective evidence and perhaps begun to incorporate some of it. It is also very good practice for the patient toward eventually being able to have this sort of dialogue with himself.

If two group members have similar ATs, they can be encouraged to role-play the ATs and, eventually, the rational responses together. This often helps minimize the "being on the spot" feelings that are often initially inhibiting when one person portrays his illogical thinking patterns by himself.

Many patients report that they appreciate having this structure imposed upon their problems. They find it more helpful than a more free-flowing discussion and are often able to report an appreciable decrease in their degree of unpleasant emotion. This decrease can be demonstrated to the volunteer and the other group members by rerating the degree of negative feelings following the exercise.

Another example of the externalization-of-voices technique follows:

VOLUNTEER: "The situation is that I'm finding myself closing off from people since my last relationship ended. I am feeling anxious and depressed."
THERAPIST: "How would you rate yourself on a 0-to-100 scale of depression, with 100 being the most depressed?"
VOLUNTEER: "Eighty-five percent."
THERAPIST: "And on a similar scale of anxiety?"

VOLUNTEER: "Ninety percent."

THERAPIST: "Please begin to tell us your anxious and depressing thoughts about the situation, using the 'you' voice."

VOLUNTEER: "You've become cold and hard and no one will ever get through to you again."

THERAPIST AND/OR GROUP: "I may be feeling a bit more reluctant to get involved now that I've been hurt, but that doesn't mean I'll always feel this way."

VOLUNTEER: "If you let down the wall you've built, others will just take advantage of you again."

THERAPIST AND GROUP: "I don't know that that is true. If it is, I may have to work on the ways in which I make myself vulnerable to others. It doesn't mean I have to give up relationships from here on out."

VOLUNTEER: "If anyone really gets to know you, they'll reject you."

THERAPIST AND GROUP: "There is nothing inherently bad or unlovable about me. Others have cared about me in the past. If I do have some problems in relating to intimates, I can work on them both inside the group and on my own. I don't have to be perfect to be in a satisfactory relationship."

VOLUNTEER: "Not wanting to be with other people means you'll be alone and lonely forever."

THERAPIST AND/OR GROUP: "I'm allowed to have a period of recovery after losing someone I cared very much about. It's natural to be protecting myself after experiencing so much pain. This doesn't mean I'll be recuperating forever. I don't have a crystal ball, and its unlikely that I've just lost the last 'love of my life.'"

THERAPIST: "Now lets turn it around and let you (the volunteer) play the more reasonable voice while the group, the other leader, and I role-play your most negative thoughts."

The process is now reversed, with the therapist and group speaking in the second person in an accusatory manner while the volunteer defends himself with the rational responses. After the reversal, the following inquiry can take place:

THERAPIST: "Where would you rate yourself now on a 0-to-100 scale of depression, with 100 being the most depressed?"

VOLUNTEER: "Fifty."

THERAPIST: "And on a similar scale of anxiety?"

VOLUNTEER: "Forty-five."

If there is little or no change in the degree of negative emotion, a discussion can ensue to examine whether or not the ATs were the most relevant ones to the negative emotions and/or what rational responses might be more productive. Patients should be reminded that they are unlikely to find the new thoughts they are articulating totally believable this early, but that just being able to conjure them up is an important first step toward eventually incorporating them in their new thinking style.

A homework assignment will be given that allows for more practice in developing rational responses for one's own set of cognitive distortions.

Homework Assignment

A homework sheet containing the following assignments is explained and distributed.

1. Divide blank NCR paper into two vertical columns. On the left side write any ATs that result in negative emotions during the week. On the right side, write the rational thoughts that counter the negative cognitions (10 to 20 ATs recommended).
2. Practice BRR once daily.
3. Practice DMR once daily, concentrating on specific problem areas of the body.
4. Consult personal goal sheet to prepare for individual midway evaluation session next week.
5. Contact buddy.

Feedback to Therapists

The therapists request feedback on the day's session from the participants, focusing particular attention on their reactions to the externalization-of-voices role-playing technique.

Personal Reminder Form

The Personal Reminder Forms are distributed. Group members are asked to complete them before leaving the group and to return one copy to the therapists.

HOMEWORK ASSIGNMENT—SESSION 6

1. Divide blank NCR paper into two vertical columns. On the left side write any ATs that result in negative emotions during the week. On the right side, write the rational thoughts that counter the negative cognitions (10 to 20 ATs recommended).

---

2. Practice BRR once daily.
3. Practice DMR once daily, concentrating on specific problem areas of the body.
4. Consult personal goal sheet to prepare for individual midway evaluation session next week.
5. Contact buddy.

INDIVIDUAL SESSION/MIDWAY
EVALUATION – SESSION 7

OVERVIEW

Attendance Taking, Homework Review, and Completion of A/P Sheets
Answering Questions on Homework Assignments or Past Sessions
Collection of A/P Sheet but Not Other Materials
Discussion of Past Objectives for the Relaxation and CBT Modules
Discussion of Other Objectives
Review of Goals for Assertion and Problem-Solving Modules
Feedback to Patient
Homework Assignment
Feedback to Therapist
Personal Reminder Form

Materials Needed:
    1. A/P sheet (Appendix 6)
    2. Individual Goal Sheet (Appendix 5)
    3. Blank NCR papers
    4. Personal Reminder Form (Appendix 10)

INTRODUCTION TO SESSION 7

In this session each group member meets individually with the group leader with whom he had met in the screening session. The intent is to review the progress each participant has made in reaching the goals developed in the screening session. The sessions can be scheduled for 30 to 60 minutes. Obviously some of the sessions will have to be held at other than regularly scheduled group meeting times.

SESSION 7

Attendance Taking, Homework Review, and Completion of A/P Sheets

The administrative tasks are performed by the individual together with the group leader, as they are in the group session.

The homework assigned at the previous session included (1) daily practice of BRR; (2) daily practice of DMR, with specific attention to body areas which have thus far been resistant to the relaxation procedure; and (3) continued work on cognitive restructuring, using the double-column technique (on NCR paper).

Answering Questions on Homework Assignments or Past Sessions

Actually, the entire session may be viewed as an opportunity to raise questions and also to foster a heightened understanding of what work has yet to be done by the patient in attaining his goals. The therapist can make suggestions that will aid the participant in reaching a moderate level of mastery of the previously introduced skill areas—relaxation and cognitive restructuring.

Collection of A/P Sheet but Not Other Materials

Discussion of Past Objectives for Relaxation and CBT Modules

At this point the goal sheet is referred to as a record of the patient's past objectives for the relaxation and CBT modules. Patient and therapist assess the progress toward these goals that has already been made; they also consider what remains of the initial problems.

An example of a persisting problem relating to relaxation follows:

Problem: Specific muscle groups are still difficult to relax.
Recommendation: These difficult muscle groups most commonly include the forehead, neck, jaws, and shoulders or upper back. Frequently, merely repeating the original instructions for that specific muscle group is sufficient to relieve the problem. The repetition in a private session can be useful in clarifying what might have been confusing or in simply emphasizing the importance of

practice. The patient is told that if no relief is obtained from an additional week of practice using these same tensing instructions, then the therapist may suggest special DMR instructions such as (1) discontinuing all tensing for that muscle area, that is, only relaxing the specific area; (2) more frequent practice, with particular attention to that body part; or (3) looking for environmental cues that are consistently paired with the tension, letting them be a signal for relaxation.

Case Example

A patient in the evaluative session reported muscular tension emanating from the back of his neck. He was cautioned not to strain too hard when practicing but to practice more frequently, carefully monitoring the SUD level (see Session 2) in his neck as well as his overall bodily SUD level. Time was spent to help locate the environmental cues that seemed to signal the onset of the feeling of tension. Following this, ways of restructuring his schedule were suggested so as to (a) avoid the occurrence of these cues and/or (b) turn them into cues for relaxation. Specifically, this patient reported significant increases in muscular tension whenever his office phone rang. It was recommended that he take steps to have his calls screened and to make his direct line inaccessible to outside callers. In addition, he was instructed to use the sound of the phone as a signal for relaxation. Thus, in practice sessions he was told to pair the imagined sound of the phone with his final relaxed state.

Problems relating to the area of cognitive change are usually addressed by using an externalization-of-voices procedure and the strong suggestion for written homework to build on this effort. Frequently, the problem area for cognitive restructuring has not been previously raised by the patient; often, it relates to personally embarrassing topics like a past incident of failure (e.g., being fired) or sexual functioning (e.g., difficulty or the fear of difficulty in being aroused).

Discussion of Other Objectives

Any new goals the patient may have developed for the two previous modules are also discussed, with strategies suggested for those parts of the new goals not yet achieved.

Review of Goals for Assertion and Problem-Solving Modules

In preparation for the second half of the group program, the patient's goals for the assertion and problem-solving modules are reviewed. Revisions of the previously developed goals are made and new ones are recorded.

Feedback to Patient

At this point in the evaluative session the therapist has the opportunity to give important information to the patient on the patient's interpersonal style. For many patients and therapists, this is a pleasant and positive experience. In other instances, where there are significant problems in interpersonal functioning, the enjoyable aspects will be missing, but the opportunity for growth on the part of the patient is priceless. The area for feedback might relate to very fundamental, objectively verifiable traits such as body posture. However, the troublesome traits may be in the realm of the subjective, which would be harder to document and, perhaps, more difficult to change.

Obviously, the patient's receptivity to this intervention is critical here and is often a function of how the therapist presents himself and his message. The therapist *is* being judgmental, there is no denying this fact. The critical issue is that there is no malice intended, and this point must be emphasized. The following is a sample dialogue:

> John, there is something I want to tell you about your functioning in the group which I regard as very important. I've discussed this with Carolyn [the co-therapist] and we both feel it's important for you to hear this. There are many things about you which are extremely likable—for example, your engaging smile and ready wit. However, we have both noted that your tendency to talk at great length, often on topics unrelated to the group agenda, leads people to stop listening to you closely and to resent your presence in the group somewhat. I am telling you this not to cause you unnecessary pain or to punish you but so that we might spend some time now discussing this aspect of your functioning in the group and to attempt to work on some strategies for change.

Often patient and therapist will work out a strategy for change that will call for additional private meetings to work on these troublesome interpersonal issues. On occasion the co-therapist is met with as well. Rarely has such an intervention been anything but positive for both the patient and the group.

Homework Assignment

The assignment from this session contains the potential for many individualized efforts in the areas of relaxation, cognitive restructuring, and interpersonal functioning. In addition, the patient is asked, in preparation for next session's new module (assertion training), to (a) read the first four chapters of Manuel Smith's book *When I Say No I Feel Guilty* and (b) contact his buddy in the course of the week.

Feedback to Therapist

The therapist now solicits feedback from the patient on his reactions to the session—both positive and negative—as well as any suggestions the patient might have to improve the evaluative session. This is also a particularly good opportunity to request feedback from the patient to how the therapist is coming across interpersonally—whether the therapist might be exhibiting certain styles of functioning that might be inhibiting his effectiveness either with this patient or the group in general. If the patient should offer feedback at this point, it is an excellent opportunity to model appropriate behavior on how to accept criticism.

Personal Reminder Form

As in prior sessions, the patient is asked to fill out a Personal Reminder Form. In this evaluative session in particular, there may be much for the patient to write down; time should be allowed for this possibility.

HOMEWORK ASSIGNMENT—SESSION 7

1. Individualized assignment for
   Relaxation _____

   _____

   Cognitive restructuring _____

   _____

   Interpersonal functioning _____

   _____

2. Read Chapters 1 through 4 of Manuel Smith's *When I Say No I Feel Guilty.*
3. Contact buddy during the week.

THE ASSERTION-TRAINING MODULE —
SESSION 8

OVERVIEW

Attendance Taking, Homework Review, and Completion of A/P Sheets
Answering Questions on Homework Assignments
Collection of Relaxation Log, A/P Sheet, and CBT Homework
New Relaxation Material
Introduction to Assertiveness Training
Homework Assignment
Feedback
Personal Reminder Forms

Materials Needed:
1. A/P sheet (Appendix 6)
2. Individual Goal Sheets (Appendix 5)
3. Relaxation Practice Log (Appendix 8)
4. Components of Assertive Behavior (Appendix 22)
5. Scripted Assertive Scenes (Appendix 23)
6. Canned situations for assertion (Appendix 24)
7. Assertive Behavior Log (Appendix 25)
8. Personal Reminder Form (Appendix 10)
9. Homework Assignment sheet

INTRODUCTION TO THE ASSERTION-TRAINING MODULE

Sessions 8 through 11 are devoted to the teaching of the assertion skill (aside from a brief refinement of the relaxation skill in Session 8).

Assertiveness training requires considerable role playing, hence one of the major tasks of the leaders is to foster a willingness to play roles. This is done through successive approximations: first by supplying a script, then by providing selected universal topics, and finally by inviting personal examples. In addition, constructive feedback is emphasized as a communication skill and several specific assertiveness skills are introduced and practiced.

Although assertiveness is the central focus of this module, cognitive restructuring is regarded as an integral part of this skill. The absence of assertion—either through passivity or agression—may be a function of distorted thinking as well as a behavioral deficit. Both problem areas are addressed.

The reading of Smith's book, conscientiously completed logs, and buddy contact are regarded as important components in the honing of assertiveness skills.

INTRODUCTION TO SESSION 8

This session is the basic introduction to assertiveness training. After explaining and illustrating the last refinement of the relaxation skill—whole-body relaxation—the leaders attempt to present the concept of assertion and to distinguish it from passivity and aggression through role-playing examples. One key concept is the idea that everyone has assertiveness deficits; we can all benefit from recognizing them and from practice.

The roles played by dysfunctional thinking and behavioral deficits in giving rise to nonassertive behavior are presented. The multiple components of assertive behavior are stressed in discussion and illustrated through role plays. The concept of constructive criticism is explained, illustrated, and emphasized. The session ends with the emphasis on setting personal assertiveness goals for homework and on recording this progress.

SESSION 8

Attendance Taking, Homework Review, and Completion of A/P Sheets

One of the therapists takes attendance while the other distributes the A/P sheets. The homework assignment from last session is repeated as an aid to filling out the A/P sheet. The assignment was as follows: (1) practice individualized instructions for interpersonal functioning, cognitive restructuring, and for both the BRR and DMR with completion of the questions about the Relaxation Practice Log, (2) read four chapters of the Smith book, and (3) contact buddy once in the course of the week.

Participants are requested to complete the A/P sheet, subtracting appropriate deductions from the initial deposit (if any).

Answering Questions on Homework Assignments

The therapists ask for any questions on or responses to any of the homework assignments. Participants are encouraged to discuss any problems they may be having with the present skill level of DMR, with the readings on assertion, or with the cognitive restructuring module.

Collection of Relaxation Log, A/P Sheet, and CBT Homework

Once all problems and questions have been discussed, one therapist collects all materials that will not be needed later in the session. For this session that would include the Relaxation Practice Log, the A/P sheet, and the CBT homework. The other therapist can briefly peruse the assignments and A/P sheets for a general impression of the compliance level of the group as well as the degree to which the various skill levels have been achieved.

New Relaxation Material

Whole-body relaxation. In Session 2 one of the leaders demonstrated whole-body relaxation. In less than 10 seconds, he reported feeling "appreciably more relaxed" while merely sitting quietly with his eyes open, staring at the opposite wall. At this point in their training, after six weeks of practice, the group is ready to do their own "whole-body procedure"—that is, to relax all muscle groups simultaneously without focusing on specific body parts.

The instructions are to:

> Sit comfortably in your chair, monitor your breathing, noting the greater sense of relaxation each time you exhale. Now imagine, if you will, that you are being covered in relaxation, as if it were some viscous material— like paint—and you are having it poured over you from head to toe. As you are covered by this imaginary substance, all the tension disappears and the relaxation takes over.

The therapists explain the concept of whole-body relaxation (i.e., relaxing one's entire body simultaneously, focusing on each muscle group in turn). One therapist introduces the demonstration, stating that the other therapist "will now show you the end point of this relaxation training. He will relax himself in seconds, and the fact that he is using the technique will be imperceptible to any observer." An analogy can be made to the slapstick cartoon where one comic character breaks an egg over another's head and the egg flows uniformly down the victim's body.

The utility of this method is reiterated, emphasizing its advantages over other relaxation techniques. One main advantage is that the technique can be used in almost any situation. Unlike many other relaxation procedures, it does not require one to close one's eyes or to be lying or sitting in any particular position. In addition, one doesn't need a quiet environment or solitude. This is one of the few, if not the only, relaxation technique that can be employed while engaging in normal workaday activities.

Group members are instructed to practice whole-body relaxation at least once daily and also to begin developing a cue system letting them use it periodically throughout the day to decrease their overall daily tension level. An example of this cueing would be for someone who suddenly finds himself inexplicably tense at work to program in whole-body relaxation every time he walks to the water fountain or every time he sharpens his pencil. Any cue which is frequent enough to provide periodic relaxation as a tension reducer may be used. Only when discovering a problem in obtaining effective relaxation results should the patient return to the more basic relaxation instructions of the tension–relaxation sequence.

Introduction to Assertiveness Training

Reactions to Reading the First Four Chapters of "When I Say No I Feel Guilty"

Group members are invited to comment on the content of this book and to ask any questions that might have arisen in the course of reading the assigned chapters. Strong positive and negative reactions to the Smith book are not uncommon, but prolonged discussion is discouraged because of the large amount of material to be covered in this session.

Defining Assertion and Differentiating It from Aggression and Nonassertion

The group leaders begin the introduction to assertiveness training by defining the alternatives to assertive behavior. These are aggressive behavior at one extreme and nonassertive behavior at the other.

Aggressive behavior is described as denying another's rights and feelings by blaming, name-calling, and other behaviors that hurt the other person and tend to elicit defensiveness.

Nonassertive behavior is described as denying one's own rights by not standing up for oneself or not expressing one's feelings. It can also include such indirect communication that misinterpretations can easily occur.

Assertive behavior is characterized by violating neither one's own rights nor those of others. It is expressing one's own feelings and preferences in a direct, honest, and appropriate manner. Assertive behavior shows respect for the other's feelings and facilitates two-way communication.

After describing assertion, nonassertion, and aggression, the therapists proceed to role-play all three behaviors in one situation. An example of a situation that could be used is "You have just been examined by your physician and given a prescription for an unfamiliar medication. You have not been given a diagnosis. The physician appears to be in a hurry. You would like a diagnosis and an explanation of his decision to prescribe the particular drug."

Once the scene is described, the therapists can alternate role-plays of aggressive, assertive, and nonassertive modes of responding to this problem situation.

The following are examples of what could be included in each model of behavior:

Example 1. An aggressive patient might respond thus: "I'll never come to see *you* again. I've never been treated so poorly. Any doctor worth his salt would have sat down with me and explained all this. You should be drummed out of medicine. Don't try to explain. I've had it with you."

Example 2. A nonassertive patient might either say nothing or speak in such an indirect fashion that his requests and comments are easily overlooked. For instance:

PATIENT: Doctor, I have to bother you but I was wondering, uh, well, uh, what is causing my chronic sore throat?

DOCTOR: Don't you worry about that. Just take these as prescribed and you'll feel much better. Call me if there are any problems.

PATIENT: Well, I'd kind of like to know what, uh . . .

DOCTOR: I really have to go now. If you're not feeling better by the time your prescription runs out, please call me. Have a good day.

PATIENT: You, too. Goodbye.

Example 3. An assertive patient might handle this situation in the following way:

PATIENT: Doctor, I would like to know about my diagnosis and also something about the medication you've prescribed.

DOCTOR: Just take these pills until they're all gone and you'll be fine.

PATIENT: I really feel uncomfortable taking unfamiliar medication and also about not really knowing what is causing this sore throat. I would greatly appreciate it if you would take a few more minutes with me to answer my questions.

Any situation can be used for this section, which can easily illustrate the three different behaviors. An alternative to the therapists role-playing these vignettes is to have the group members act out the different behaviors. Advantages of this method are that (1) the therapists can get a measure of the group members' understanding of the differences among the behaviors; (2) it is an easy entree into having the group members give each other feedback, which is an integral part of the assertion training module; and (3) any mistakes that are made by the participants while role-playing can be useful as a teaching device in illustrating the differences among the behaviors. Disadvantages of this method are that: (1) group members may be reluctant to role-play this early in the assertiveness training sequence; (2) they may either feel that the role-playing assignment is too difficult, and therefore anxiety-producing, or too easy, and therefore demeaning; and (3) it may be too time-consuming to have the members volunteering and then role-playing, and the examples may not be as clearly differentiated from each other as they might be if the therapists did the role playing themselves. The group leaders can weigh the advantages and disadvantages above and can use either method, depending upon their preferences and their assessment of the group members' skill level.

Describing the Role of Assertion in Preventing or Lessening Dysfunctional Emotions

Assertion training can be described to the participants as another method of decreasing anxiety and depression. Assertive behavior is often incompatible with anxiety and depression and can sometimes be an effective antidote for these emotions or a good way of preventing them.

Examples can be given of individuals who became depressed because they were not expressing their feelings or not actively pursuing their life goals. Taking an active approach by increasing one's assertive behavior can often result in alleviating a dysphoric mood. Research has shown that assertion is negatively correlated with depression (Shaffer, Shapiro, Sank, & Coghlan, 1981) and that assertiveness training can significantly improve one's self-concept (Lange & Jakubowski, 1976).

Anxiety can also be diminished by assertive behavior. Strong feelings of anxiety are often incompatible with being appropriately assertive. Unassertive behavior, on the other hand, is frequently associated with headaches, gastric disturbances, backaches, and other symptoms of tension (Jakubowski-Spector, 1973).

Illustration of the Cognitive-Restructuring and Skills-Training Components of Assertion

For the purpose of this introductory explanation, assertive behavior can be broken down into two basic components. The first major aspect of assertion is one's cognitions; the other is one's level of skill in behaving assertively. The cognitive component of assertion includes the specific thoughts or thinking style which would prevent one from being appropriately assertive. Typical examples of distorted thinking that often results in lack of assertion are (1) "If I say how I really feel, they won't like me and that would be unbearable." (2) "My opinion isn't really important enough for me to speak up." (3) "I shouldn't be having these feelings, so I should just keep them to myself." Thoughts such as these are very effective inhibitors of being direct, open, and honest with others. It is important that participants be made aware of this bridge between the cognitive restructuring and assertion modules. They can be encouraged both in the session and through homework assignments to continue to make use of their ability to challenge dysfunctional thinking.

The other component of assertion is the actual skill level that is necessary to appear appropriately assertive. Assertive behaviors in most instances include: (1) eye contact, (2) facial expression, (3) gestures and body posture, (4) voice tone, inflection, and volume, (5) content, and (6) timing. A list of these behaviors (see Appendix 22) can be given to each participant while one group leader explains how they relate to assertion. An example of this explanation follows:

Eye Contact. Eye contact is extremely important in presenting an appropriately assertive image. Lack of eye contact can give undesirable messages such as "I'm very anxious" or "I don't believe what I'm saying."

Voice Tone. The most assertive message can be lost by delivering it in a too quiet voice. This gives the impression of insecurity and/or fear. On the other hand, a message that is delivered in too loud a voice can distract the listener and/or put him on the defensive.

Posture. An appropriately assertive position can vary from situation to situation. However, as a general rule one should aim for holding one's body errect in a posture that is neither rigid (connoting tension) nor too relaxed (which may appear disrespectful or not serious).

Facial Expression. A common problem that can dilute one's assertive message is a facial expression that is not congruent with what one is saying. For example, to smile while saying "That makes me angry" gives the listener a mixed message and fails to convey the intended message. This inconsistency is often born of a desire to protect oneself in case the listener finds the content of the statement unacceptable, but it can serve as a self-fulfilling prophecy.

Timing. The most appropriately designed assertive statement can be wasted if one chooses an inappropriate time to present it. The boss is unlikely to respond favorably to a request for a raise, no matter how well the request is executed, if he is approached as he is scurrying to tie up loose ends before a big meeting.

Content. All other appropriate assertive behaviors can be undermined by message content that sounds either blaming and aggressive or meek, mild, and passive. The content of an assertive statement ideally is precise, descriptive, and straightforward. Further suggestions and techniques to improve content will be presented in the following sessions.

Discussion of Assigned Reading and Review of Individual Goals Established for Assertion Module

Group members are asked to give their reactions to the assigned reading in *When I Say No I Feel Guilty.* Responses often vary from "It's really helpful and perfect for me" to "It's boring, repetitive, and unreasonable." The participants with the latter impression are encouraged to glean from the book what they can and to use it as a "consciousness raiser" to aid them in becoming more aware of situations in which they would like to be more assertive.

At this point, the individual goal sheets are returned and each member is asked to talk about his goals for the assertion module. These goals may be revised at this time in light of the previous discussion, the reading in the group, and prior experiences. Encouragement is given for making these goals specific, behavioral, and measureable, so that it will be obvious to the patient when he has accomplished one or all of them.

Role Playing of Vignettes Illustrating Common Assertion Problems, Including Instructions on Giving Each Other Feedback

There are three levels of role playing that can be used initially in a group format, depending upon the skill level and sophistication of the participants. The first level is to have scripts prepared so that participants begin by merely reading an assertive response to a particular situation. This is the most elementary level of role playing and would be appropriate for participants who are reluctant to role play or who are unable to arrive at any semblance of an assertive response without a great deal of help. (See Appendix 23 for two such examples.)

The second level is role playing an assertion problem that has already been created by the group leaders. The participants are asked to behave assertively in these "canned" situations. This level is often less threatening than dealing with one's own problem in front of the group and yet does serve the purpose of easing the participants into role playing and giving them practice with the techniques they will be learning. (See Appendix 24 for several of these set scenes.)

The third level is for group members who are feeling more self-confident and/or eager to work on their own individual problems. These participants can begin by role-playing personal examples from their own lives. They would begin by stating the problem, setting the scene, and informing their "co-role-player" as to how he should react. Participants can either choose another group member to role-play with them or one of the group leaders. Another aid to reluctant role-players is to have them describe the situation but have two others in the group—either leaders or participants—role-play it first. This is often an easy first step to role-playing one's own particular situation.

Once a role-play has taken place, the group leaders present a model for giving feedback before any comments are made. A reminder sheet containing the following elements of constructive feedback is distributed:

1. Give positive feedback first, telling the role-player what he did well, for example, "Your eye contact was very good."
2. Rather than criticize, make suggestions for what could be changed next time, for example, "Your voice could be a bit louder."
3. Be specific about behaviors, for example, "This particular hand gesture (demonstrate) could be distracting."

4. Give examples of how something could be said differently, for example, "Your husband may hear 'unproductive' as a buzz word and be offended. You may want to talk about 'not accomplishing as much as we'd like.'"

Assertive Behavior Log (ABL). Throughout the assertiveness module, participants will be asked to keep track of their progress in recognizing challenges to their assertiveness and their relative success in meeting their challenges. The ABL provides a format for tracking progress and noting areas requiring emphasis and skill building (See Appendix 25).

Homework Assignment

Assignment sheets are distributed outlining the following homework:

1. Practice whole-body technique for DMR once per day.
2. Practice differential relaxation technique for DMR once per day.
3. Practice BRR once per day.
4. Read up to half of *When I Say No I Feel Guilty* (Chapters 5 to 8).
5. Contact buddy once during the week.
6. Attempt new assertive behaviors and complete one copy of Assertive Behavior Log (ABL).

Feedback

Group members are asked to talk about what they found helpful this session and what changes they'd like to make in the format of future sessions.

Personal Reminder Forms

The personal reminder forms are distributed. Group members are asked to complete them before leaving and to return one copy to the group leaders.

HOMEWORK ASSIGNMENT—SESSION 8

1. Practice whole-body technique for DMR once per day.
2. Practice differential relaxation technique for DMR once per day.

---

3. Practice BRR once per day.
4. List 5 to 10 ATs that inhibit assertiveness, generating rational responses to them (on NCR paper and to be handed in).
5. Read up to half of *When I Say No I Feel Guilty* (Chapters 5 to 8).
6. Contact buddy once during the week.
7. Complete one copy of Assertive Behavior Log (ABL).

THE ASSERTION-TRAINING MODULE – SESSION 9

OVERVIEW

Attendance Taking and Completion of A/P Sheets
Answering Questions on Homework Sheets
Explanation of Specific Assertion Techniques
Role-Playing Vignettes Using Specific Assertion Techniques
Guided Feedback
Generation of Individual Goal-Oriented Scenes for Role Playing the Following Session
Homework Assignment
Feedback to Therapists
Personal Reminder Form

Materials Needed:
1. Relaxation Practice Log (Appendix 8)
2. Assertive Behavior Log (Appendix 25)
3. Videotape recording and playback equipment (optional)
4. Personal Reminder Form (Appendix 10)
5. Homework Assignment sheet

INTRODUCTION TO SESSION 9

In this session group members are exposed to the specific assertion techniques of the broken record, fogging, and disarming. Following their definition (which also appears in the reading assignment), actual experience in the use of these techniques is provided. The participant may use a personal example, or a vignette can be supplied. The intent is to help the patient recognize situations where assertion can be used to provide specific tools to be employed in the situations. As in Session 8, feedback is carefully monitored to be kept constructive. The session closes with an emphasis on employing these skills outside the session and on bringing in the troublesome situations as grist for the next session's mill.

SESSION 9

Attendance Taking, Homework Review, and Completion of A/P Sheet

The administrative tasks are performed as in previous sessions. The homework assigned for Session 9 included (1) daily practice of BRR; (2) daily practice of DMR—whole-body and differential relaxation; (3) reading the second quarter of *When I Say No I Feel Guilty*; (4) listing 5 to 10 ATs that inhibit assertiveness and their corresponding rational responses (on NCR paper); (5) one buddy contact; and (6) attempt new assertive behavior and completion of one Assertive Behavior Log (ABL).

Answering Questions on Homework Assignment

At this point group members are encouraged to ask questions regarding the homework assignment and any part of the material they might feel requires further explanation. This can include the reading assignment that was to have been completed for this session. Questions and comments about the cognitive components inhibiting assertion are encouraged.

Explanation of Specific Assertion Techniques

Although the major task of the assertion module (indeed, of all modules) is to assist each participant in reaching his individual goals as specified on his goal sheet, a parallel goal is to teach a broad range of skills that may increase the participant's abilities in a wider range of problem areas. The techniques that will be introduced (i.e., broken record, fogging, and disarming) may not necessarily be used by the participant for all his specific goals. However, the group exercise facilitating the use and recognition of these techniques should enhance the participant's comfort in the frequent use of assertive skills.

The specific techniques that follow are defined by the leaders and examples are role-played. When necessary, additional examples can be supplied by therapists or participants.

The Broken Record

One of the easiest to learn but also most controversial assertion technique is the *broken-record technique* (Smith, 1975). This method of asserting oneself involves *repeating one's major point again and again without becoming angry or blaming*. It is often very useful with strangers who are trying to avoid taking responsibility for their error or are trying to deflect one from one's goal.

Group members may have a negative reaction to this technique because they may see it as both transparent and infuriating to the person with whom they would be dealing. These objections may be answered by pointing out that one has the option of choosing when to use each technique and that the broken record may be chosen to deal with particularly trying situations in a business or other impersonal encounter where the participant is willing to be transparent or infuriating.

The following is an example of how the broken-record technique was used by a group member and reported as a homework assignment:

> The Foreign-Pizza-Person Episode
> After work on Friday, I called up the local pizza place and ordered our standard TGIF pizza: a medium-size deep-dish combination to go. The man taking orders on the phone did not speak English very well. I told him that I wanted a "combination pizza" but couldn't recall this pizza parlor's lingo for same. He told me that it was either a "supreme" or a "super-supreme," and I asked what the difference was between the two. We then had a five-minute conversation trying to reach an understanding about what was actually *on* a "supreme" versus "super supreme." I ended up ordering the supreme sans "pork topping." When I arrived at the pizza parlor, my pizza was ready; but when the cash register person rang up the total, it came to almost three dollars more than we usually pay. I asked about the discrepancy and was told that I had not ordered a *combo* pizza but rather a regular, plain cheese pizza with *extra* peppers, onions, pepperoni, mushrooms, and cheese—in other words, a "supreme" pizza without the "pork topping."
>
> Calling up my previous hand-to-hand combat assertiveness training, I refused to pay the extra money and inquired about the pizza parlor's policy on deletions and substitutions from combos. I was told that deletions and substitutions could be made.
>
> At that point, the foreign-speaking person who had taken my order originally entered into the fray and attempted to force me to

pay the greater amount, alleging the mistake was mine and not his. I did the old broken-record routine, but when I decided I wasn't going to get anywhere because of the language problem, I asked to speak to the manager. This time the broken record worked. He relented and charged me the lesser amount.

Example of our dialogue:

ME: I ordered a combo pizza without the pork topping and was charged three dollars extra. I am not willing to pay the extra amount.

MANAGER: What you really had there was a plain cheese pizza with substitutions.

ME: This is the same pizza I always order. I'm not willing to pay three dollars extra for a mistake I didn't make.

MANAGER: By not having the pork topping, you're not having the "supreme," therefore you don't get the special price.

ME: I inquired and was told that it is this pizza parlor's policy to permit deletions and substitutions on combination pizzas. I do not intend to pay the extra three dollars.

MANAGER: Very well. You can pay the lesser amount. However, next time please be certain to specify that you are deleting from a "supreme" rather than adding to a "plain."

ME: Thank you.

Fogging (Smith, 1975)

Fogging is also an effective though frequently misunderstood technique which involves *finding something you can agree with when someone is attacking you verbally.* The same technique is called *disarming* by Burns (1980b). Both fogging and disarming help "cool" another's anger by not fueling it with defensive or attacking statements. By initially defending yourself, you are more likely to make the attacker feel misunderstood or challenged and driven to come up with more and more evidence to justify his anger. Agreeing with any small part of what has been said makes you sound accepting of the angry person's feelings and can mollify him to the point where he is able and willing to work on the problem.

This technique has been criticized for suggesting that the assertive person might actually agree with the terrible and unfounded statements that are being made. On the contrary, the suggestion is to search for the grain of truth in the attacker's barrage and agree with it rather than choosing an obvious error and beginning with a counterattack. An example of the fogging or disarming technique follows:

ATTACKER: That shirt looks terrible on you. You never dress well when we go to visit my friends.

ATTACKED: This isn't my favorite shirt either. What don't you like about it?

ATTACKER: It's wrinkled and the color is bad for you. You have no taste in clothes and you embarrass me.

ATTACKED: I'm sorry that you've felt embarrassed. Choosing clothes isn't my strong suit. Perhaps you'd like to help me choose what I wear tonight.

ATTACKER: Yes, I would. I'm sorry I flew off the handle. Thanks for putting up with me. Maybe we can go shopping together this weekend.

The conversation reported above could have gone very differently had "the attacked" responded defensively and/or attacked in kind. For example:

ATTACKER: That shirt looks terrible on you. You never dress well when we go to visit my friends.

ATTACKED: You have your nerve. I think it looks fine. You're no beauty queen yourself.

ATTACKER: What are you trying to do, undermine my self-esteem? I should have never married such a jerk.

ATTACKED: Well, don't worry—no one else would have you. But if you think you can do better than me, go ahead and try.

ATTACKER: Maybe that's just what I'll do. (Slams door as she walks out.)

Role-Playing Vignettes Using Specific Assertion Techniques

Group members can now be given the option of using either canned vignettes or their own real-life situations to practice the broken-record and fogging or disarming techniques. Some groups or some individuals may be very enthusiastic about getting into their own problem areas, while others may feel reluctant and prefer to use impersonal situations for their initial practice sessions.

Topics for canned vignettes can include the following situations:

1. You have been asked to supervise another employee and find that you are dissatisfied with his work. This employee is very defensive. It is your goal to tell the employee about the problems in a way that does not blame or belittle him but also allows you to carry out your supervisory responsibilities effectively.
2. A friend has invited you on a picnic. However, as time progresses, you find that she is expecting you to do most of the cooking and preparation. Your goal is to maintain the friendship and, if possible, retain the plans for the picnic, but only if the labor is shared.
3. For personal reasons you have decided not to eat or drink at a party you are attending. Your hostess is making a valiant effort to get you to consume something. It is your goal not to offend her yet not to change your resolve about not eating or imbibing.

4. You have just had dinner with a new acquaintance and would like to end the evening now. The acquaintance would like to continue talking with you at your home. Your goal is to say goodnight promptly at your door without hurting or alienating the other person.

5. The person with whom you live has not been doing his share of the household chores. Your goal is to arrange for a more equal distribution of labor without causing hard feelings or an unpleasant scene.

These situations and others can be written on slips of paper and chosen randomly by all of the group members or just by those who choose not to role-play their own real-life situations.

Whether he is using a canned scene or another of his own choosing, each role player is asked to "set the stage" by describing where the role play should take place, deciding who will play the other part and stating how that person should behave. Role players are asked to practice using a combination of the broken-record and fogging or disarming techniques in these vignettes whenever possible.

Videotaping (Optional)

If videotape equipment is available, it can be very useful in helping patients see themselves as others see them. This can be particularly helpful for patients who are unaware of distracting, unattractive, or otherwise inappropriate mannerisms (see the discussion of guided feedback that follows).

Patients should be given the option not to be videotaped if they have strong objections. Those with inhibiting mannerisms, however, might well be encouraged to take advantage of this seldom available type of feedback.

Guided Feedback

After each vignette has been role-played, the participants are encouraged to give the role players feedback on the behavioral components of assertive behavior. The recommendations for giving constructive feedback (see Session 8) are reiterated and the therapists model appropriate commentary as well.

The group members may need to be prodded to give feedback at first. However, the modeling and calling on participants should be sufficient to encourage this important aspect of assertiveness training.

It is also frequently useful to have one patient who has given helpful feedback to role-play how he may have improved his assertive performance in the situation. The co-therapists can do this as well, illustrating a change in behavior that would be more functional or effective for the patient. In addition, role reversal (i.e., having the participant role-play the antagonist—the person with whom he wishes to interact) can assist the role player in determining what the antagonist might be feeling, what he might say, or how he might behave. It can also result in increased empathy for the other individual, which can be an aid in preventing behavior that is inappropriately aggressive or lacking in compassion.

If someone else has modeled for the patient, or once he has taken the "counter role," the patient can be given another chance to try his hand at attempting to improve his performance.

Videotaping (Optional)

If videotape is being used, the entire vignette can be replayed at once, with everyone making notes for commentary later, or the machine can be stopped each time someone wants to give positive feedback or to recommend a change. Alternatively, it is often helpful to ask for comments before the tape is replayed. Using the videotape is usually more time-consuming than unassisted feedback, but it is also often much more complete and much more powerful.

Generation of Individual Goal-Oriented Scenes for Role Playing the Following Session

At this point the group members may or may not have used the group to work on their own personal assertion problems. It is usually much easier to get group members to think of personal examples at the end of a group where they have been focusing on these issues than it is to have them volunteer at the beginning of a new session. Therefore, it is recommended that the leaders ask for examples from the participants' lives which they might want to work on in the next week's session. This will help to save time the following week to coax and encourage group members to volunteer for role playing. The participants can then simply be reminded at the outset of next session of their specific problem areas and role playing can begin almost immediately, using both new and previously taught techniques. Those who may be unable to volunteer a problem area at the end of the group can be requested to work at finding one as a special homework assignment.

Homework Assignment

Assignment sheets are distributed outlining the following homework:

1. Practice whole-body technique for DMR once daily, accompanied by the pleasure and/or mastery scenes.
2. Practice differential relaxation techniques for DMR once daily.
3. Practice BRR once daily.
4. Complete relaxation log for items #1, 2, and 3 above.
5. Read up to three-quarters of *When I Say No I Feel Guilty* (Chapters 9 and 10).
6. Contact buddy once during the week.
7. For role playing, bring in at least one situation in which you'd like to be more assertive.
8. Attempt new assertive behaviors and complete one copy of the Assertion Behavior Log.

Feedback to Therapists

Group members are asked to give the therapists their reaction to this particular session (e.g., what they found helpful and what they would like to change for future sessions).

Personal Reminder Form

The personal reminder forms are distributed and group members are asked to fill them out and to return one copy to the leaders before leaving the session.

HOMEWORK ASSIGNMENT—SESSION 9

1. Practice whole body technique for DMR once per day accompanied by the pleasure and/or mastery scenes.
2. Practice differential relaxation techniques for DMR once per day.
3. Practice BRR once per day.
4. Complete relaxation log for #1, 2, & 3 above.
5. Read up to 3/4 of *When I Say No I Feel Guilty* (Chapters 9 and 10).
6. Contact buddy once during the week.
7. Bring in at least one situation for roleplaying in which you'd like to be more assertive.
8. Attempt new assertive behaviors and complete one copy of assertion behavior log.

THE ASSERTION-TRAINING MODULE —
SESSION 10

OVERVIEW

Attendance Taking, Homework Review, and Completion of A/P Sheets
Answering Questions on Homework Assignment
Collection of Relaxation Logs, A/P Sheets, and Other Written Assignments
Discussion of Reading Assignment for Session 10
Explanation of Specific Assertion Techniques
Role Playing of Preplanned, Individual Goal-Oriented Vignettes Using Specific Assertion Techniques
Guided Feedback
Generation of Individual Goal-Oriented Scenes for Role Playing the Following Session
Homework Assignment
Feedback to Therapists
Personal Reminder Form

Materials Needed:
1. A/P sheet (Appendix 6)
2. Relaxation Practice Log (Appendix 8)
3. Personal Reminder Form (Appendix 10)
4. Homework Assignment sheet

INTRODUCTION TO SESSION 10

Session 10 introduces two additional assertion techniques ("I" messages and active listening). Their practice is encouraged when personal situations are role-played by various group members. This session is primarily devoted to working on individual assignments employing specific techniques whenever possible and building group cohesion as an impetus for setting and accomplishing outside assignments. Once again, feedback is carefully monitored for its constructiveness and participants are encouraged to commit themselves to outside assignments and future performances (role playing) at the next session.

SESSION 10

Attendance Taking, Homework Review, and Completion of A/P Sheets

The administrative tasks are performed as in previous sessions. The homework assigned in Session 9 included (1) practice BRR once daily; (2) practice DMR twice daily, once using differential relaxation, once using whole-body relaxation with scenes; (3) read up to three-quarters of *When I Say No I Feel Guilty;* (4) bring in one situation for assertiveness role playing during this session; (5) contact buddy once during the course of the week; and (6) attempt new assertive behaviors and complete one copy of the Assertion Behavior Log (ABL).

Answering Questions on Homework Assignment

The group is now invited to pose questions about the homework assignment as well as about any material from prior sessions, including the cognitive restructuring and relaxation modules.

Collection of Relaxation Logs, A/P Sheets, and Other Written Assignments

All written materials are collected except the Assertion Behavior Log (ABL), which may be referred to during the course of the session.

Discussion of Reading Assignment for Session 10

In the course of reading the companion text for the assertion module, many questions arise about the quality of the writing or the intentions of the author. The therapists are well advised to deflect these questions into topics for *brief* group discussions and to avoid being placed in the position of being staunch defenders of the author. In almost every group, one can expect to find those who will vilify an author and those who will swear by him. Little is gained from discussing the book *as a whole*; much can be gained from discussing the merits and applicability of specific techniques. In this session, as in Sessions 9 and 11, we will discuss such techniques (though they are not all derived from the Smith book).

Explanation of Specific Assertion Techniques

As in the last session, the group members are introduced to additional specific assertion techniques: "I" messages and active listening. Both these techniques are adapted from Gordon's *Parent Effectiveness Training* (1970) and both are valuable aids to assertive communication.

The concept of "I" messages is important in the content as opposed to the behavioral component of assertive behavior. By learning to use "I" messages appropriately, group members can communicate their feelings to others without causing unnecessary defensiveness, anger, or hurt feelings. An "I" message contains an objective description of the other's behavior and the tangible effect it has on one's own life. The following is an example of an "I" message: "I get very upset [statement of feeling] when you arrive late for dinner [behavioral description] because I put a lot of energy into meal preparation; when I have to serve the food cold or overdone, all my efforts seem to have been in vain [tangible effect on one's life]."

Gordon distinguishes "I" messages from "you" messages by their content and effects upon the listener. "You" messages contain blaming and or labeling statements that can alienate or anger the recipient. The "I" message above can be restated into a "you" message as follows: "You're always late for dinner. You're inconsiderate and selfish. You can make your own meals from now on."

"I" messages are more likely to result in increased understanding and better communication, while "you" messages can often result in misunderstanding, poor communication, and bitter arguments.

The group leaders can further illustrate the differences between "I" and "you" statements by role-playing the same situation twice, once with "I" statements and once with "you" statements. In the example that follows, one leader can play the shoe salesman and the other can play the customer.

Situation: A customer in a shoestore is presented with a pair of shoes he very much wants. However, the shoes are two different sizes.

"You" message: What kind of a store is this? You certainly can find the proper mate to this shoe. You're not trying. You've no business working here if you can't accomodate your customers.

"I" message: I'm really frustrated because I've looked all over town for these shoes and now that I've finally found them, I discover that the size is mismatched. Could you please look in the back one more time to make certain that there's not another mismatched pair in another box?

Salesclerk's potential response to "you" message: I've already told you there are no other shoes. I've looked and I'm not looking again. You can either take these shoes or look elsewhere. I don't have to listen to your accusations.

Salesclerk's potential response to "I" message: I can understand how you feel. I'm doubtful that I'll be able to find the mate to the shoe you want, but I'll give it another try. If I can't find it, I'll try our other stores to see if they have it.

Another technique that facilitates effective and responsible communication is active listening. Active listening is a method by which the listener can let the speaker know that what he is saying is being heard. The technique includes listening closely to what is being said and repeating back to the speaker a paraphrase or summary of the message received. This method of communicating has several advantages. First, it can be an important preface to an assertive statement. In a discussion, especially about sensitive issues, it is very important for the speaker to feel that he is being understood before he is ready to receive an assertive response. A second benefit is that misunderstandings can be cleared up rapidly if the content of the message is restated and the sender then has the opportunity to correct any misinterpretation.

An example of active listening follows. Speaker 1 (the employee) will be giving a message and Speaker 2 (the employer) will use the active listening approach.

SPEAKER 1: I feel that I do a lot of work around here and it never gets recognized. I haven't gotten a raise or even a pat on the back in a long time and I feel like quitting.

SPEAKER 2: It sounds as though you're feeling as though the job hasn't been too rewarding lately.

SPEAKER 1: That's right. It's really been frustrating and makes me wonder what I'm doing here.

SPEAKER 2: You feel it's become so disappointing to you that you're actually thinking of resigning.

Speaker 1: Well, I'm not certain that I would go that far, but I wanted you to hear how disheartened I've become.

As this exchange shows, active listening is not parroting the other's words but rather rephrasing what has been said in order to demonstrate one's understanding of the content.

In *Feeling Good* (1980), Burns discusses similar techniques using the terms *inquiry* and *empathy*. These methods are particularly useful in dealing with another's anger. When confronted with an angry onslaught, Burns recommends (1) "inquiry" (i.e., inquiring about the specifics of what has caused the anger) and (2) "empathy" (i.e., demonstrating an understanding of and sympathy for the other person's point of view).

In the following example, Speaker 1 (the husband) will give an angry message, and Speaker 2 (the wife) will respond, first by using inquiry and second by displaying empathy.

Speaker 1: You are always spending time with friends, but when I need your attention you're always too busy. We don't have a marriage anymore. We're just roommates and not good roommates at that.

Speaker 2: What have I been doing or saying that makes you feel as though I'm not giving you enough attention [inquiry]?

Speaker 1: You're never home when I want to do things with you, and when I try to talk to you when you do get home, you say you're too tired.

Speaker 2: I can see how you would get the idea that I'm more involved in other things. I guess I'd feel lonely too if you were doing that to me [empathy].

Speaker 1: I think you would, too. I'm feeling lonely and hurt and fearful that our marriage is disintegrating.

The techniques of "inquiry" and "empathy" can be very effective in helping to dissipate rage as well as allowing the angered party to calm down sufficiently to hear the other viewpoint. Following this, Burns recommends using his "disarming" technique, which as been described in Session 9.

Role Playing of Preplanned, Individual Goal-Oriented Vignettes Using Specific Assertion Techniques

At the conclusion of Session 9, the participants were asked to generate specific examples of personal problem areas that could be role-played in this session. These situations were written down by one of the therapists in that session. Those who did not volunteer situations at the end of Session 9 were asked to come up with a situation or situations as homework. The therapists then ask for brief descriptions of these homework situations as well.

The directions for this section are to make use, whenever possible, of the specific assertiveness techniques described earlier in Session 10 ("I" messages and active listening) as well as in Session 9 (fogging, disarming, and broken record) in role-playing the personal examples of the group members.

Videotaping is quite helpful in encouraging the learning and practice of these new skill areas as a medium of accurate recall and nonbiased feedback, but it is not essential. However, videotaping *per se* can also be inhibiting to the group members, as they become more self-conscious and less willing to take risks. This problem with inhibition also applies to those giving feedback who can feel extraneous or superfluous vis-à-vis "The Machine," which knows and can tell all.

There is usually not sufficient time to have each member work on his personal example in this session. However, each member should have an opportunity to describe his problem situation. Simply describing the situation can provide a form of verbal rehearsal that facilitates future action. The description also represents a kind of public commitment to change for the patient, a subtle pressure on him to take action on his own behalf.

Although it is most likely that all the situations will not be able to be worked on in this session, each group member should have an opportunity to be a part of at least one role-played situation—either as protagonist or foil.

The therapists stress the use of the various techniques both before and even during the role play (through subtle and not-so-subtle coaching). Following the patient's description of the situation and in anticipation of the "action," the therapists inquire of and give prompts to the patient about which techniques could be utilized; the foil, especially when reverse role-playing, can also practice these skills. An example follows:

THERAPIST: OK, John, to summarize, you've been having these problems with your roommate, Jack, for some time now. He refuses to clean up the dinner dishes and "borrows" with no offer to replace the food you've purchased for yourself.

JOHN: Essentially, that's right, and I want him to be aware that I'm wise to him and don't like it.

THERAPIST: And you'd also like him to change in the future?

JOHN: Yeah.

THERAPIST: What I'd like you to do, then, is this role-played scene—and you listen, too, Paul, because you'll be the recipient of this assertion and may, if we reverse roles, be using them yourself on John. I'd like you to use "I" messages in telling your roommate about how you feel and to be ready with active listening for any explanation he might give. Fogging or disarming and the broken-record technique might be used here, but let's see how the scene progresses.

The therapists should feel free to interrupt the scene at critical points to suggest the use of the newly learned skills at appropriate points. Naturally, interruptions can be overdone and should be kept to a minimum (one or two brief interventions per five-minute scene).

Guided Feedback

As in Sessions 8 and 9, group members are given feedback. Positive comments are shared first, followed by constructive suggestions. All group members are encouraged to participate in this exercise, which is also a way of practicing new assertive skills.

Generation of Individual Goal-Oriented Scenes for Role Playing the Following Session

As in the last session, group members are asked to generate situations from their own past, present, or future that they can use the following week to role play the techniques being taught. These plans for next week's session are carefully written down by the members.

Homework Assignment

1. Practice DMR twice daily, once doing whole-body DMR with the pleasant and mastery scenes and once using differential relaxation.
2. Practice BRR once daily.
3. Complete relaxation log for daily practice.
4. Complete *When I Say No I Feel Guilty* by reading Chapter 11 and the Summary.
5. Contact buddy once during the week.
6. For role playing, bring in at least one situation in which you'd like to be more assertive.
7. Attempt new assertive behaviors and complete one copy of Assertion Behavior Log (ABL).
8. List 5 to 10 ATs that inhibit assertiveness, generating rational responses to them (on NCR paper and to be handed in).

Feedback to Therapists

The therapists again request that the group members give them feedback on today's session, emphasizing what they found helpful and what they would like to do differently in future sessions.

Personal Reminder Form

The Personal Reminder Forms are distributed. Group members are asked to complete them and to return one copy to the leaders before leaving the session.

HOMEWORK ASSIGNMENT—SESSION 10

1. Practice DMR twice daily, once doing whole-body DMR with the pleasant and mastery scenes and once using differential relaxation.
2. Practice BRR once daily.
3. Complete relaxation log for daily practice.
4. Complete *When I Say No I Feel Guilty* by reading Chapter 11 and the Summary.
5. Contact buddy once during the week.
6. For roleplaying, bring in at least one situation in which you'd like to more assertive.
7. Attempt new assertive behaviors and complete one copy of Assertion Behavior Log (ABL).

THE ASSERTION-TRAINING MODULE —
SESSION 11

OVERVIEW

Attendance Taking, Homework Review, and Completion of A/P Sheets
Answering Questions on Homework Assignment
Collection of Homework Assignments, A/P Sheets, and Relaxation Logs
Discussion of Assigned Reading
Use of Cognitive Restructuring Techniques to Aid in Promoting Assertive
    Behavior in More Emotionally Difficult Situations
Explanation of the Use of Conflict Resolution
Role-Playing of Remaining Individual Goal-Oriented Vignettes
Guided Feedback
Homework Assignment
Feedback to Therapists
Personal Reminder Form

Materials Needed:
    1. Relaxation Practice Log (Appendix 8)
    2. A/P sheets (Appendix 6)
    3. Assertive Behavior Log (Appendix 25)
    4. Video equipment (optional)

INTRODUCTION TO SESSION 11

This final assertion session follows the same outline as past sessions. Some new material (conflict resolution) is introduced but the strongest emphasis is on employing these new assertion skills in the personal situations brought in by each participant. There is a shift backward to the cognitive restructuring module as a means of addressing the most resistant of personal assertion challenges. As in past sessions, role playing is the major patient activity in the session. Patients are urged to work on their toughest personal problems and, as they leave this module and begin the last section of the program (problem solving), to commit themselves to chart a course of change.

SESSION 11

Attendance Taking, Homework Review and Completion of A/P Sheets

The homework assigned in Session 10 included (1) twice daily practice of DMR, once using the whole-body technique and once using differential relaxation; (2) once-daily practice of BRR; (3) completion of relaxation log; (4) completion of *When I Say No I Feel Guilty;* (5) attempt new assertive behaviors and completion of one Assertive Behavior Log; (6) one buddy contact; (7) for role-playing during the next session, bringing in at least one situation where increased assertion would be desirable; and (8) listing 5 to 10 ATs that inhibit assertiveness, generating rational responses to them.

The administrative tasks are accomplished as in the past sessions.

Answering Questions on Homework Assignment

As in past sessions, questions are encouraged. Some are dealt with briefly, some are deferred for private consultation (rarely), some are used as lead-ins to the new material, and others are deferred for later explication and/or practice during the session (e.g., role playing; see below).

Collection of Homework Assignments, A/P Sheets, and Relaxation Logs

This is done as in prior sessions, leaving out the Assertive Behavior Logs, which may be taken up later in the session.

Discussion of Assigned Reading

The reading of *When I Say No I Feel Guilty,* as assigned, should be completed by Session 11. A general discussion of the various techniques introduced by Smith is often useful. Group members will frequently discuss their utility, how they have actually put them to use, and any inhibitions they might have about employing them. This last issue (inhibition) serves as a useful introduction to a discussion of the role of irrational or automatic thinking as it prevents appropriate assertive behavior.

Use of Cognitive Restructuring Techniques to Aid in Promoting Assertive Behavior in More Emotionally Difficult Situations

As was discussed in Session 8, nonassertive behavior can be a function of deficient skills, distorted cognitions, or both. The preceding three sessions have discussed and worked on the former. The new material for this session addresses the central role that cognitions can play in facilitating or inhibiting assertive responses.

Although some of the earlier exercises contained elements requiring both cognitive and behavioral change, the emphasis was clearly on the latter. However, as the subjective level of difficulty increases for the patient—as he is asked to meet greater challenges—the shift is toward an emphasis on cognitive change.

The homework called for generating a situation or situations that the patient would wish to work on in the coming week and listing cognitions that would inhibit assertion. In this section, the therapists illustrate the role of cognitive deficits or distortions as inhibitors by calling upon group members and asking for the ATs (or IBs) that may have hindered success in the assignment. An example follows:

JIM: I'm always getting a call from my mother each Sunday evening since I left home to get married. That was 12 years and three kids ago. And I resent the intrusion. It's as if I having nothing better to do than be home for her call or to give a detached running account of sore throats, spelling tests and the size of my prize zucchinis. Susie and I haven't been able to escape a call in years; not even when we were away on vacation!

THERAPIST: You seem to have very strong feelings about this, yet you've allowed it to go on for many years. What seems to prevent you from doing something about this? (*This serves as the inquiry into the cognitive distortions that hinder an assertive response.*)

JIM: Well, I . . . I guess I'm afraid that I'd crush her if I suggested that she not call me so often or that she not ask me those silly questions.

THERAPIST: That sounds like a catastrophizing error to me as well as the fortune-telling and mind-reading error. Could it be that she's as tired of this phone call ritual as you are and is afraid that she might hurt *your* feelings (or crush *you*) if she didn't call?

JIM: You know, Doc, I actually considered that when writing out this homework. It just might be so. I only wish that I could raise the issue with her.
THERAPIST: Well, that's a real change ! Why not work on the cognitive part of that difficulty as homework, using the double-column technique. What we can do now is to practice the dialogue you'd be using once you have to come to terms with the inhibiting cognitive distortions.

A role play would follow.

The process is a simple one. First, be sensitive to the presence of cognitive distortion in the subjectively more difficult assertiveness assignments. Second, inquire after the precise ATs, suggesting alternative self-statements (rational responses). Third, use the skills already established in past sessions in assigning homework and, fourth, work on the behavior that had been inhibited by the dysfunctional thinking, thus facilitating the actual accomplishment of the patient's self-generated task.

Explanation of the Use of Conflict Resolution

Conflict Resolution as a term was introduced by Gordon (1970) as a method for parents and children to use in resolving their differences without acrimony and power struggle. The same technique is very useful between adults, as well and has been used to resolve conflicts among business people, to develop labor contracts and to expedite out-of-court legal settlements.

Conflict resolution is basically the use of a problem-solving approach to deal with interpersonal differences. Problem solving as a coping skill for individuals will be dealt with more fully in Sessions 12 and 13. As an assertion technique between equals, however, conflict resolution is a very effective follow-up to active listening, "I" messages, inquiry, and empathy. Once the other person's viewpoint is understood and both agree as to what the problem is, one can then say "Let's brainstorm," "What might be a solution that would satisfy you?" "Let's try to think of several ways we could solve this problem," and so on. Rather than giving a command, making a demand, or being manipulative, one can suggest a "workable compromise" (Smith's label for this same assertive technique). Conflict resolution or the workable compromise have the advantages of offering more creative solutions, preserving equality and fairness in the outcome, and creating a sense of cooperation among the parties involved.

The following is an example of the use of conflict resolution to deal with a potentially difficult situation. The husband in this situation is telling his wife that his children from his first marriage will be visiting for the summer. The wife finds this particularly stressful due to the disruption it will cause in her own life and also because she is not particularly fond of the children. A potentially acrimonious discussion was prevented in this case by the use of "I" messages, active listening, and conflict resolution.

A sample of their discussion follows:

HUSBAND: Honey, the kids want to spend the summer with us again.

WIFE: That upsets me because I have a lot of things planned for this summer, and you'll also recall that the girls and I don't get along that well ["I" message].

HUSBAND: You do have a lot to do this summer and I realize that being with the girls that much is unpleasant for you [active listening]. Is there any way we could make their visit more palatable for you [conflict resolution]? It's extremely important for me to have this time with them ["I" message].

WIFE: I guess that if you feel that strongly, we could try to think about what could make it better for me [conflict resolution]. One thing would be that you could entertain them by yourself sometimes, so I could have more time to myself.

HUSBAND: That would be fine with me. How often would you want me to do that?

WIFE: Well, at least once or twice a week.

HUSBAND: That sounds reasonable. What else would help?

WIFE: I think that it would be good for me to get away for a week. Perhaps I could visit some friends in New York or go see my family.

HUSBAND: I'd hate to see you go, but I can understand how that would be good for you. It would also give me more time to get reacquainted with the girls. I could also, while you're here, be more helpful around the house, because I realize two extra people make a lot more work.

WIFE: I really appreciate your trying to make this easier for me. If we do all that we've said, perhaps this summer can work out to everyone's satisfaction.

Role-Playing of Remaining Individual Goal-Oriented Vignettes

Group members are asked to apply any relevant assertion skills they've learned to date in role-playing actual situations in their lives. Because this is the last session in the assertion module, the participants are encouraged to choose situations for role playing and discussion which are more demanding emotionally and/or more difficult behaviorally. Some cognitive restructuring may have to be applied before certain role plays are attempted. This can be done quickly by having the fellow group members generate reasonable responses to any distortions that are uncovered. To aid in the use of other newly learned techniques, the group leaders can suggest, if appropriate, the use of "I" messages, empathy, inquiry, conflict resolution, and so on during the actual role-playing sessions.

Guided Feedback

As in past sessions, group members are encouraged to give each other constructive feedback on the content and style of their assertive communication. These final role plays often involve very important and troubling areas in the participants' lives. At this point constructive feedback from both the group members and the leaders is critical in giving the role player an indication as to how his message may be viewed by significant others in his life. Those whose role plays continue to seem too aggressive or too nonassertive should be given the feedback and encouraged to do more reading and more practicing (in less crucial situations) before attempting a potentially damaging encounter.

Homework Assignment

1. Practice DMR twice daily, once using whole-body relaxation, alternating both scenes, and once using the differential relaxation technique.
2. Practice BRR once daily.
3. Complete Relaxation Practice Log.
4. Complete one Assertive Behavior Log.
5. Contact Buddy.
6. Review your goal sheet in preparation for the problem-solving module.

Feedback to Therapists

The group members are asked to discuss what they felt was accomplished in the day's session and any changes they'd like to make in future sessions.

Personal Reminder Form

All participants are requested to complete the Personal Reminder Form for the day's session and to give a copy to the leaders.

HOMEWORK ASSIGNMENT—SESSION 11

1. Practice DMR twice daily once using whole-body relaxation, alternating both scenes, and once using the differential relaxation technique.

2. Practice BRR once daily.
3. Complete Relaxation Practice Log.
4. Complete one Assertive Behavior Log.
5. Contact buddy.
6. Review your goal sheet in preparation for the problem-solving module.

THE PROBLEM-SOLVING MODULE –
SESSION 12

OVERVIEW

Attendance Taking, Homework Review, and Completion of A/P Sheets
Answering Questions on Homework Assignment
Collection of Relaxation Log, A/P Sheets, and Other Written Assignments
    from Session 11
Introduction to the Problem-Solving Module
Explanation of the Problem-Solving Process
Example Role-Played by Therapist
Discussion of Individual Goals
Homework Assignment
Feedback to Therapist
Complete Personal Reminder Form

Materials Needed:
    1. AP sheet (Appendix 6)
    2. Relaxation Practice Log (Appendix 8)
    3. Problem-Solving Homework Sheet (Appendix 26)
    4. Example of Completed Problem-Solving Homework Sheet (Appendix
       27)
    5. Homework Assignment sheet
    6. Personal Reminder Form (Appendix 10)

INTRODUCTION TO THE PROBLEM-SOLVING MODULE

In this module we attempt to tie up the loose ends. The participants
had many goals to be reached in the relatively short span of 15 sessions.

All of these goals will not have been achieved at this point or even at the conclusion of the 15th session. This last group of sessions is designed to teach a new skill that will enable the participants to make better use of each of the preceding modules. Problem solving attempts to provide a structure for the consideration of and formal attack on problems that resist ready solutions. Within the context of teaching them how to solve problems, the group members will also be reexposed to the many ways in which the first three modules (relaxation, cognitive restructuring, and assertion) might be employed to reach remaining goals.

This module provides another opportunity to build group cohesion, and it often yields very positive results. Members are asked to combine forces in devising multiple alternative solutions to each other's problems. Often constructive interpersonal feedback is offered in the context of solving related problems. In addition to teaching the actual skill of problem solving, we often see a real sense of purpose in the participants as they come to terms with the fact that they have the requisite tools with which to tackle what had once seemed to be insurmountable problems.

INTRODUCTION TO SESSION 12

In this session the specific components of problem solving are presented and explained. An example of a problem is given and the solution process is role-played by a therapist. Members are asked to describe their particular goals for this module and to consider what other areas of their lives might reasonably be included here. (Often this module is least understood at the screening sessions, so participants are encouraged at this point to reconsider what might have been their very limited expectations for this module.) Once again, a homework form is emphasized in this module. The Problem-Solving Homework Sheet (Appendix 26) is integrated into the skill-building process. Emphasis is again placed on homework assignments and their completion.

SESSION 12

Attendance Taking, Homework Review, and Completion of A/P Sheets

The administrative tasks are performed as in previous sessions. The homework assigned in Session 11 included (1) review of goal sheet in preparation for the problem-solving module; (2) practice BRR once daily;

(3) practice DMR twice daily, once using the whole-body relaxation with both scenes and once using the differential relaxation technique; (4) complete Relaxation Practice Log; (5) call buddy once during week; (6) complete one additional Assertive Behavior Log.

Answering Questions on Homework Assignment

Group members are encouraged to ask questions about the material covered to date. This includes the relaxation, cognitive restructuring, and assertion modules.

Collection of Relaxation Log, A/P Sheet, and Other Written Assignments from Session 11

The A/P records, relaxation logs, and other written assignments from Session 11 (i.e., cognitive restructuring double-column sheets and Assertive Behavior Logs) are collected.

Introduction to the Problem-Solving Module

This new module, the last of the sequence, is designed to focus upon those areas in the patient's life that continue to place him in turmoil. It is designed to (1) help him put these difficulties in perspective and (2) provide a means of resolving these and future dilemmas. The skills and attitudes introduced in the preceding modules will provide many of the essential ingredients used in this module. The problem-solving module will use the preceding skill areas to develop approaches designed to resolve these challenges to effective living. The continued presence of these persistent, unresolved problems creates discomfort in itself and can lead to troubling psychological difficulties such as mood disorders.

In a complex society, there are always problems in living. However, the development of a learning set (Harlow, 1949) allows for a more positive, direct approach to the resolution of life problems. This approach can help to prevent dysfunctional mood and behavior disturbances that might otherwise arise.

Explanation of the Problem-Solving Process

Problem solving can be broken down into a series of steps. The serial nature is not necessarily an accurate representation of how individuals always go about solving problems. Often, in the process of problem resolution, steps will be omitted, repeated, and reversed. However, it is suggested that when a person faces a perplexing problem, one with potential psychological ill effects, he will do well to follow the problem solving process outlined below. When confusion, dysphoria and anxiety set in, any systematic approach (there are variations on this problem-solving sequence) can ease the way to a favorable solution.

General Orientation

The eight-step approach is preceded by a preliminary general orientation which is essential to developing a solution-oriented learning set. The orientation calls for the patient to understand and expect that he, like most people, will experience a number of problems over time. He has not been singled out and need not view himself as any more or less subject to the misfortunes of living. In addition, he is prepared to recognize problems as they arise, not to avoid or deny them. This does not imply that he should take precipitous action but rather that he ought to set into motion the steps of problem resolution that follow.

1. Problem Identification. This first step calls for the patient to appreciate the background of the problem: its history of recurrence and of attempted resolution as well as its relevant historical variables. The patient is then called upon to define the problem precisely, acknowledging any complicating factors; is this a conflict between a goal and an obstacle or a goal and another goal? Following this precise formulation of the problem, the patient proceeds to the following steps.

2. Goal formation. The patient responds to the question: What would signify the resolution of the problem?

3. Generation of Alternatives. Following the recognition of the goal, the patient is asked to brainstorm alternatives, to generate as many alternative solutions to the problem as possible. This is done in an uncritical, unjudgmental way, with an emphasis on quantity and the building of one suggested alternative on another.

4. Evaluate Alternatives. After brainstorming solutions, the patient turns to evaluating the likely consequences of the courses of action given in step 3. These alternatives are evaluated on both positive and negative dimensions with the task of determining an ultimate rating (a scale of 1 to 5 is used).

5. Decision Making. Based on the evaluations performed in step 4, the patient decides on the most likely alternative(s) to resolving his problem.

6. Verification. The patient now addresses the question: Is the alternative selected in step 5 likely to lead to the resolution of the problem?

If not, the patient is called upon to return to step 3 and repeat the process from there. If the answer is yes, he then proceeds to:

7. *Preparation for Implementation.* In this critical step the patient identifies the course of action necessary to implement the action identified in step 5 and verified in step 6. Occasionally this step will involve another process of systematic problem solving, so as to develop the *means* to resolve the original problem.

8. *Implementation and Outcome.* The last step specifies the outcome of the course of action taken in terms of the problem and goal as defined in the foregoing process.

Example Role-Played by Therapist

After the explanation of the eight-step problem-solving process, one therapist presents a role-played illustrative problem as per the outlined steps (see Appendix 27 for abbreviated handout). An example follows: "I have just broken up with my boyfriend and want to get out socially and to meet other men."

1. *Problem Identification:*
    a. *Background (specify):* "Charles and I were dating for four years on and off, the last year with much turbulence. He finally called off our relationship last week."
    b. *Detail Problem Situation:* "I am very shy and actually stayed in the relationship to avoid having to search for another man. I hate typical meeting places or rituals."
2. *Goal Formation* (how you'll know when you've solved the problem): "I want to increase my opportunities to meet eligible men."
3. *Generation of alternatives:* Brainstorm as many situations as you can without censoring them:
    a. Take a university course.
    b. Join the "Y."
    c. Go to church singles functions.
    d. Join a ski club in winter, beach house in summer.
    e. Call your friends and let them know you're available.
    f. Speak with Charles and ask him to tell *his* friends that you're available.
    g. Call up some eligible man at work and invite him out for a drink.
4. *Evaluate Alternatives* in terms of their probable consequences:

Pros	Cons	Rating effectiveness (1 = least; 5 = most)
a. "I could meet someone ambitious."	"I dislike evening courses; my job is too demanding."	2
b. "I like athletics."	"Most activities are not coed."	1
c. "I am religious but have neglected that part of me; there is an active singles group at my church."	"I may have to introduce myself as a newcomer."	4
d. "There are plenty of singles at these activities."	"These singles are social butterflies, they're very competitive."	2
e. "I'll be 'set up' if it works; it requires little initiative."	"It's doubtful that they have any 'live ones' that they aren't cultivating themselves."	3
f. "Charles has some male friends."	"Charles would never help me, and his friends are jerks."	1
g. "Joe is very attractive; I've had my eye on him for months."	"I can't imagine myself summoning up the nerve."	3

5. *Decisionmaking.* Based on evaluation rating (above), choose the most likely alternative(s): Option (c), go to church "singles" functions, is the most likely effective alternative.

6. *Verification* for appropriateness of selected alternatives: Is this alternative likely to reach your goal?

7. *Preparation for Implementation:* What steps are necessary to implement the chosen alternative?
   a. I can call my church to obtain the singles schedule.
   b. I can make certain that I do not book myself up for these evenings.
   c. I can buy some appropriate clothes.
   d. I can call my pastor and let him know I'll be coming.

8. *Implementation and Outcome.* Specify outcome in terms of identified problem. Though I didn't meet "Mr. Right," I suppose I've met several of his friends and am attending church functions regularly with them, hoping they will bring him along some evening. My circle of friends has widened and I am invited to parties where I have an increased chance of meeting an eligible man.

Following this illustration of the problem-solving technique, the group is invited to make comments on the procedure and to discuss its range of applicability. This serves as a natural lead-in to:

Discussion of Individual Goals

Using their goal sheets, group members are asked, in turn, to discuss their individual goals for this module. This module often is the most difficult in terms of eliciting goals. In part the paucity of goals is attributable to the fact that problem solving is taken up last. Often, by this time, most problems have been addressed (successfully or unsuccessfully) in past modules, consequently patients risk repeating themselves (i.e., using past problem areas) or may have a very small list. Encouraging the members to brainstorm (step c, *Generation of alternatives*) often helps in obtaining a greater number of goals and in motivating the participants to use the module appropriately.

Homework Assignment

The assignment for the coming week includes the following: (1) become aware of additional problems for the current module and bring list next time; (2) complete one problem-solving form; (3) bring in one problem to be worked on in the next session; (4) BRR once daily; (5) DMR twice daily, once doing the whole-body relaxation technique using both scenes, once doing differential relaxation; (6) complete relaxation log; and (7) contact buddy once in the course of the week.

Feedback to Therapist

As in past sessions, the feedback of the group members is solicited.

Complete Personal Reminder Form

As in past sessions, the patients fill out the Personal Reminder Form before leaving the session.

HOMEWORK ASSIGNMENT—SESSION 12

1. Become aware of additional problems for the current module and make a list for next time.

2. Complete one problem-solving form.
3. Bring in one problem to be worked on in the next session.
4. BRR once daily.
5. DMR twice daily, once doing the whole-body relaxation technique using both scenes, once doing differential relaxation.
6. Complete relaxation log.
7. Contact buddy once in the course of the week.

THE PROBLEM-SOLVING MODULE –
SESSION 13

OVERVIEW

Attendance Taking, Homework Review, and Completion of A/P Sheets
Answering Questions on Homework Assignment
Collection of Relaxation Log and A/P Sheet
Group Exercise in Identifying Problems for the Problem-Solving Module
Group Exercise in Generating Alternatives for the Problems Brought in by
    Participants
Brief Preview of Closing Sessions
Homework Assignment
Feedback to Therapists
Personal Reminder Form

Materials Needed:
    1. A/P sheet (Appendix 6)
    2. Relaxation Practice Log (Appendix 8)
    3. Problem-Solving Homework Sheet (Appendix 27)
    4. Homework Assignment sheet
    5. Personal Reminder Form (Appendix 10)

INTRODUCTION TO SESSION 13

This second and last problem-solving session is mostly devoted to group exercises employing the problem-solving skill. Most group members should have the opportunity to have their particular problem worked on by the group. Often there will be common themes, allowing groups of two or three participants to "own" the problem (i.e., to define it and evaluate the proposed alternatives). The session closes with an emphasis on commitment to change and the resolve to use the various skills already learned in the program to implement this change.

SESSION 13

Attendance Taking, Homework Review, and Completion of A/P Sheets

The administrative tasks are performed as in previous sessions. The homework assigned in Session 12 included the following: (1) become aware of additional problems for this problem-solving module and bring a list to the next session; (2) complete one Problem-Solving Homework Sheet (Appendix 26); (3) bring in one problem to be worked on in session 13; (4) practice BRR once daily; (5) practice whole-body DMR once daily, using both practice scenes, and practice differential DMR once daily; and (6) call your buddy once during the week.

Answering Questions on Homework Assignment

Group members are encouraged, at this point, to ask questions about the material covered in the past, but with particular emphasis on the last session's material (e.g., problem solving).

Collection of Relaxation Log and A/P Sheet

The completed Problem-Solving Homework Sheet is collected at the end of the session, but the problem list is not. This, it is hoped, will serve as a reminder to the patient of his unfinished business.

Group Exercise in Identifying Problems for the Problem-Solving Module

The problem-solving technique is actually quite easy to teach and relatively easy to apply to appropriate situations. The greatest challenge in this module is getting the group members to recognize problems suitable for this technique and to appreciate its value for them personally.

Appropriately enough, the method that has proved most useful in getting patients to learn when to apply the problem-solving strategy has been an application of the problem-solving format.

Participants are asked to contribute, in turn, to a list (written on the blackboard or on newsprint) of those problems where the problem-solving method could be usefully applied. The patients are encouraged to consult their own personal lists (brought in as homework), or they may use more hypothetical areas. Specificity is requested (e.g., "I want to find a roommate to help share expenses in my townhouse" is more useful than "problems with mortgage payments"). In addition, as is stressed in the brainstorming section, quantity is valued, alternatives are not censored, and the process of building responses one upon another is encouraged. A sample list follows:

List of Potential Problems Where the Problem-Solving Technique May Be Applied

1. How to get to work on time
2. How to make money in my spare time
3. How to get _____to ask me out
4. How to get my spouse to be more romantic
5. How to get my spouse to be sexually more aggressive
6. How to pay for my next vacation
7. How to get my neighbor to treat his dandelions
8. How to be more productive at work
9. How to get my daughter to do her homework
10. How to stay within my budget

This exercise is often helpful in generating increased enthusiasm about the utility of the module. Too often, it is viewed as common sense but is dismissed. It *is* commonsensical but is also too rarely applied in times of stress. The following exercise builds on the momentum generated while the group was considered the wide applicability of the problem-solving skill.

Group Exercise in Generating Alternatives for the Problems Brought in by Participants

At first by getting volunteers, then through calling upon people, the leaders ask that the problem each participant had brought in to work on as part of his homework assignment be described briefly (with necessary background) and specified in terms of a goal. The group is then asked to go through the brainstorming exercise generating as many alternatives as possible for each of the problems presented, with no effort at censoring the alternatives but with support for building on previous suggestions. The alternatives are recorded by the therapists. Following the brainstorming exercise the problem owner is asked to rate each potential solution on the 1 to 5 scale. Next, the highest rated alternatives(s) are selected (decision-making step) and evaluated as to their likelihood of solving the problem (verification step). An example follows.

GROUP MEMBER 1 (MARY): I've just discovered that my husband has a loaded revolver in his bedroom dresser. We've just gotten married, he for the first time, I for the second, and I have my two small children in the house (ages 8 and 4). I want this threat to my children's well-being removed.

THERAPIST: First, Mary, that sounds like an excellent problem to work on in this module. You were thorough—you furnished us with the problem, brief background material, and your goal. What I would like now is for each of us to think of at least one alternative to help Mary achieve her goal. Remember the emphasis is on quantity and potentially building on a preceding promising alternative. And, Mary, please don't pass judgment on these alternatives until we've completed this part of the exercise. I'll be writing as all of you speak.

GROUP MEMBER 2: Speak to your husband and tell him that you're upset and why.

GROUP MEMBER 3: Bring him the statistics about fatalities with handguns and that the victims tend to be family members.

GROUP MEMBER 4: He'll never change, hide it from him.

GROUP MEMBER 5: Rather than hiding the gun, take away the ammunition.

THERAPIST: Good, You're building on the previous alternative.

GROUP MEMBER 2: I think that you two could work this out. Discuss it. How about suggesting that the gun and shells be separate and hidden from the kids?

THERAPIST: That gives us five alternatives; we could go on for several more. But for the purposes of this exercise, we can have Mary evaluate what we've generated thus far.

MARY: Actually, these were fine suggestions. I'm satisfied to stop at five.

THERAPIST: Okay, Mary, now please evaluate the alternatives as I read them to you. Give us your positive and negative reactions as far as how they will help meet your goal. Then rate them on a scale of 1 to 5; 1 is least, 5 is most potentially effective.

MARY: Fine, I'm ready.

THERAPIST: The first alternative was to speak to Hank and tell him that you're upset and what you're upset about.

MARY: That would be beneficial in opening up the lines of communication. I won't feel closed off from him but, on the negative side, he may just call me an hysteric (he does that a lot), and it certainly wouldn't get rid of the gun.

THERAPIST: And your rating?

MARY: I'd give it a 2.

THERAPIST: The second alternative is to present Hank with the gun statistics about how accidents with guns show that it's the gun owners or their families who tend to be the victims of these weapons.

MARY: The positive aspects of communication are in this alternative, and, in addition, I'd be having my discussion based on facts. On the negative side, I still couldn't be sure Hank would do anything about the gun. I'd give it a 3.

THERAPIST: Fine. Now the third alternative suggests that you hide the gun from Hank.

MARY: Well, I'd be certain then that the gun would be out of the house, but when Hank found out he'd be furious. Besides, it's wrong to just take away someone's property without some discussion and agreements.

THERAPIST: And how would score that alternative?

MARY: I'm afraid I'd have to give it only a 1. Sorry, Joanne.

JOANNE: That's all right.

THERAPIST: Remember we were brainstorming in step 3. No one has to feel that their alternative has to be chosen. It's a building process at that stage. How about the next alternative, taking away the ammunition?

MARY: Well, it *would* accomplish my goal of removing the danger from the house, but on the other side of the ledger, it still is taking away something of Hank's without his permission. I wouldn't want him doing that to me. I'd rate this one only slightly higher than the previous alternative, a 2.

THERAPIST: Finally, we have the fifth suggested solution of discussing the situation and making the suggestion that the gun shells be placed and hidden separately to keep them from your children.

MARY: I really like this alternative! It diminishes the danger significantly. We'll have a chance to talk it out, too. The only drawback is that I couldn't be certain that Hank would go along with my suggestion.

THERAPIST: And your rating of this alternative?

MARY: I'll give it a 4.

THERAPIST: Then, in looking at your ratings of the five alternatives, you'd choose . . . which?

MARY: The last alternative: Discuss it with Hank and suggest separating the gun and the ammunition and hiding them separately.

This exercise is designed to strengthen the problem-solving skill. Patients report that repeated use makes the procedure more automatic and more comfortable.

Brief Preview of Closing Sessions

The group is briefly prepared for the closing sessions. Sessions 14 and 15 include asking the patient to take stock of the problems and goals held prior to the screening session and to compare his position then with the position he is in now. He then addresses the issue of what steps to

1. Problem Identification
   a. Background (specify): <u>My husband had this gun prior to our recent marriage and sees it as necessary for our protection.</u>

   b. Detail problem situation: <u>My children (from a previous marriage) will be endangered.</u>

2. Goal formation (How will you know when you've solved the problem?): <u>I want the danger removed.</u>

3. Generation of alternatives (Brainstorm for as many alternatives as you can without censoring them):

   a. <u>Speak to my husband, tell him I'm upset and why.</u>

   b. <u>Tell my husband about the dangers of a handgun at home.</u>

   c. <u>Hide the gun from my husband.</u>

   d. <u>Take away the ammunition.</u>

   e. <u>Discuss the problem and suggest separating the gun from the shells.</u>

4. Evaluate alternatives in terms of their probable consequences:

	Pros	Cons	Rate potential effectiveness (1 = least; 5 = most)
a.	Promotes open communication	He'll say I'm a hysteric; danger is still there.	2
b.	Communication and facts	The danger may still be there.	3
c.	Positive action	He'd be furious; it violates my principles.	1
d.	Positive action	I'd still be violating his property rights.	2
e.	Promotes communication and positive action (by making a suggestion)	I couldn't be sure that he'd do it.	4

5. Decision making—Based on evaluation rating (step 4), choose the most likely alternative(s):

   Alternative e

6. Verification for appropriateness of selected alternative: Is this alternative likely to reach your goal? If not, return to step 3. Yes (☐)　No (☐)

It's not sure to get me to reach my goal, but Hank is reasonable and likes to please me.

7. Preparation for implementation. What steps are necessary to implement the chosen alternative?

Find a quiet moment (perhaps tonight) and broach the subject.

8. Implementation. Specify outcome in terms of the identified problem:

(Next meeting) Hank agreed with my concerns and was glad that I brought it up. He hid the gun and shells separately (but near each other in case he should need them).

FIGURE 4. An example of the problem-solving process.

take to maintain his progress and to resolve remaining problems. The homework for Session 14 is designed to help the patient answer these questions.

Homework Assignment

The patient is asked to (1) review his individual Goal Sheet, past Homework Assignment sheets, and past Personal Reminder Forms; (2) make a list of those problems yet to be solved or goals yet to be met and complete a problem-solving form for each; (3) practice BRR once daily; (4) practice DMR twice daily, once with the whole-body technique and the scenes and once using differential relaxation; (5) complete Relaxation Practice Log; and (6) contact buddy once during the week.

Feedback to Therapists

As in past sessions, the therapists solicit feedback from the participants as to what they found helpful in the session and what they would like to see changed.

Personal Reminder Form

As in previous sessions, the participants fill out Personal Reminder Forms before leaving.

HOMEWORK ASSIGNMENT—SESSION 13

1. In preparation for Sessions 14 and 15, review your Individual Goal Sheet and your past Homework Assignment sheets.
2. Make a list of the problems yet to be resolved or goals yet to be met; complete a problem-solving form for each.
3. Practice BRR once daily.
4. Practice DMR twice daily, once with the whole-body technique and with two scenes and once using differential relaxation.
5. Complete Relaxation Practice Log.
6. Contact buddy once during the week.

9

CLOSING SESSIONS – SESSION 14

PUTTING IT ALL TOGETHER

OVERVIEW

Distribution of A/P Sheets, Review of Homework, and Completion of A/P
   Sheets
Answering Questions about Homework Assignment
Collection of A/P Sheets and Processing of Refunds
Recounting of Success Experiences
Review of Remaining Problems
Feedback
Preparation for the Individual Exit Interviews
Homework Assignment
Preparation for Booster Sessions

Materials Needed:
   1. A/P sheet (Appendix 6)
   2. Individual Goal Sheet (Appendix 7)
   3. Individual goal sheet for final interview (Appendix 30)
   4. Homework Assignment sheet

INTRODUCTION TO THE CLOSING SESSIONS

The closing sessions (14 and 15) are designed to provide the participant with an understanding of how all four modules fit together and
complement each other and how their utilization can lead to a sense of
efficacy and self-control. The sessions call upon the patients to recall
their original objectives, to reevaluate their original problem areas, and

165

to take stock of themselves several months and 14 sessions later. By looking back on where they have been and what they had set as goals, the
group members have the opportunity to see—with improved perspective
and new skills—how they may have overestimated their level of inca-
pacity or set their sights too low. The original goal sheets (with their
implied problems) serve as anchor points from which to measure progress. The final sessions address how to employ what has been learned
(i.e., how to combine skills to overcome recurrent problems as well as
new ones as they arise). In addition, these sessions afford each member
the opportunity to give and receive feedback from other group members
about their group functioning and progress toward their stated goals.
Group members are invited to critique the therapy program and the therapists. They also, especially in the last session, receive detailed feedback
from one of the two leaders about their progress over the course of
treatment.

INTRODUCTION TO SESSION 14

This session begins with several usual administrative tasks, including the distribution and completion of the A/P sheets and review of
homework as well as the final tallying of the deposit monies due as a
refund. The purpose of this session is to emphasize strongly that the
modules fit together and complement one another. They were not chosen at random but rather coalesce as a formidable armamentarium that
can help patients to cope with the multiplicity of problems that they had,
still have, or might encounter in the future.

The members are again (as in the screening session) asked to
describe their presenting problems and goals, this time with an update
on their progress. Any remaining problems are discussed from a strategic
perspective—how the new skills might be brought to bear to vanquish
problems.

Last, the potentially threatening but highly valuable opportunity to
give and receive personal feedback is presented. This is the last group
session until the six-month booster, and many group members regard it
as the last opportunity to meet together and wish each other well. This
is also introduced as the opportunity to give and receive constructive
feedback about progress made and future opportunities for growth. Similarly, the therapists are able to learn about themselves and their efforts
in this constructive atmosphere. The session ends with plans for individual meetings with one of the therapists and with a discussion of the six-
and twelve-month booster sessions.

SESSION 14

Distribution of A/P Sheets, Review of Homework, and Completion of A/P Sheets

The A/P record is distributed to each group member with the request that the appropriate sections be completed for this session. As an aid in providing for accurate recording, the homework assignment from last week's session (Session 13) is repeated: (1) review goals sheets and past homework sheets; (2) determine which goals have and have not been met in the course of the group; (3) list those goals that have been met and skills that were enlisted that brought about the changes; and (4) develop a strategy for change for the most troubling problem that remains.

The group members are now asked to complete their A/P sheets. In addition they are asked to make a note of their final "balance due" from the original deposit. (This is easily done, as the A/P sheet has been designed to record the balance due each week.)

Answering Questions about Homework Assignment

Any questions regarding the homework assignment are now answered. The problem-solving forms are not collected until the conclusion of the session.

Collection of A/P Sheets and Processing of Refunds

This is preferably done with cash placed in envelopes to be distributed to everyone at the close of this session. This serves as an immediate reward without singling out anyone who has little or no deposit remaining. Otherwise checks can be mailed or held for the final session, when the patient meets individually with one of the two therapists.

Recounting of Success Experiences

Making use of the homework assignment for this session, group members are asked to describe those problems that originally brought them to the group and the success they have experienced in resolving these problems over the course of the 14 sessions. In addition, group members are asked to describe the skills they have used in overcoming these problems. Group members frequently read directly from their original goal sheet and Personal Reminder Forms, offering a commentary on each item. The group leaders press for specifics to enhance the opportunity for other members to learn from these experiences, particularly from the ways in which the various skills learned in the group have been brought to bear on specific personal problems.

Review of Remaining Problems

A major part of the session is devoted to discussing problems that persist for the group members and how their more resistant problems might be dealt with following the group's termination. The process is begun by distributing a sheet prepared by a hypothetical patient (Appendix 28) in which several resolved problems as well as several remaining problems are listed. The group reviews this worksheet together, particularly the suggested skills to be employed—singularly or in combination—in resolving those remaining problem areas. Following this group exercise, group members are often more willing to discuss their own persisting problems and to work with each other on formulating strategies to overcome remaining problems. (Appendix 29—a blank Worksheet for Remaining Problems—is useful at this point.) Again, group members are asked, in turn, to describe the most troubling problem that remains for them or one that they forsee. They are asked to begin describing a strategy for resolving this problem, and the group is called upon to lend assistance as they decide which particular skill might be appropriate and in what order. The group member is encouraged to fill in his worksheet as he discusses his particular remaining troublesome areas.

Feedback

By this point, members are familiar with each other, having seen one another through a range of circumstances and discussed some of the more intimate aspects of their lives. Provided that it is offered in a positive mode, the feedback that they could give each other on progress made and areas that remain for additional work could prove invaluable. This process is accomplished with each member receiving feedback from all other members. The leaders, especially at the outset of this exercise, will model how to give positive feedback and how to pose suggestions for continued change in a positive vein.

After this session, the therapists will have a separate session with each group member to give extensive feedback. Hence, therapist feedback in this session is designed to model appropriate statements along the dimensions of brevity, a positive nonjudgmental viewpoint, and an optimistic view of the future.

Member-to-Member Feedback

These opportunities for group members to give each other individual feedback are in many ways merely the formalization of what may have naturally occurred in the preceding sessions as members collaborated to help solve each other's problems. In addition to this collaboration, the formalized feedback session serves to call attention to the fact that this is the last in the series of sessions of group collaboration. The group members will not be meeting again for six months (the first of two booster sessions), and this feedback allows for some formal leave-taking. Positive expressions of feeling are encouraged, thus allowing the group to end on an optimistic note.

Feedback to the Group Leaders

At the close of each preceding session, group members have been asked to comment on their positive as well as negative reactions to the session just completed. The same request is make at the conclusion of this session; however, following the critique of this particular session, the scope of solicited criticism is broadened to include feedback on the entire group experience and on the group leaders themselves. In particular, recommendations for change to improve future groups are requested and the therapists demonstrate a willingness to hear comments and suggestions about the therapists' individual styles as well as how they interact as a team.

The opportunities for patient feedback have proven enormously helpful in producing ideas that eventually resulted in the refinement of this group program. The comments on the therapists' style can also encourage the therapists' growth, both individually and as a team. On rare occasions, a patient may abuse the feedback opportunity, but prompt intervention as well as assertive, self-disclosing. and disarming replies can turn less than constructive criticism into an opportunity to model some important skills to the group.

Preparation for the Individual Exit Interviews

The group leaders next explain that each member will have an individual session with one of the group leaders. This session is scheduled for approximately one week after Session 14. The purpose of this last meeting is, in part, a continuation of the give-and-take feedback procedure that has just taken place. In addition, the therapist will have greater latitude in probing for remaining issues and in formulating plans for additional treatment, if appropriate.

Homework Assignment

Group members are asked: (1) to prepare a list of areas or problems in their lives that may not have been discussed in the final group session (Appendix 30). This list will include both goals met and those not yet accomplished. Participants are asked to bring this list to their private interviews. This list is to include any items that were not brought up in this current session or which may not have been adequately discussed in the session. Once again, the goal sheets that were prepared in the screening session are suggested as a resource for this final homework assignment; (2) to continue with daily BRR practice; (3) to practice DMR twice daily, once whole body with scenes and once with differential relaxation; (4) to complete Relaxation Practice Log; and (5) to contact buddy.

Sign up sheets are next circulated to allow patients to choose preferred meeting times for their individual sessions. (See Session 15 for further discussion.)

Preparation for Booster Sessions

In preparation for the six-month follow-up session, patients are requested to keep a log of occasions on which the skills proved useful and when they did not. The patients are given a card with the date and time of the six-month follow-up session. (They will also be called one month before this date as a reminder.)

HOMEWORK ASSIGNMENT—SESSION 14

1. Prepare a list of problem areas that were not discussed in Session 14.
2. Continue daily BRR practice.
3. Continue twice daily DMR practice, once with whole-body relaxation with scenes and once with differential relaxation.
4. Complete Relaxation Practice Log.
5. Contact buddy.

CLOSING SESSIONS – SESSION 15

FINAL INTERVIEW

OVERVIEW

Orientation of Group Member to Final Interview
Review of Individual Goals and Evaluation of Progress
Formulation of Strategies to Achieve Remaining Goals
Developing Future Goals and Planning for Implementation
Therapist Feedback to Patient
Patient Feedback to Therapist
Reminder of Six-Month Booster Session

Materials Needed:
  1. Individual Goal Sheet (Appendix 30)
  2. Appointment cards with time and date of booster session

INTRODUCTION TO SESSION 15

The purpose of this session is to provide a final opportunity for the group member and one of the group leaders to deal with any issues not directly addressed or disclosed in the group setting. This session is also useful in designing individualized strategies for accomplishing any goals yet remaining or any recently formulated goals for the future. In addition, the group member and leader can together attempt to foresee any pitfalls or potential critical incidents in the future and can discuss what skills can be used at those times to cope with new and stressful situations. Finally, this session can be useful in providing additional feedback for both the patient and therapist in the evaluation of the group experience.

These sessions can be brief (30 minutes) or can last as long as an hour depending upon the setting, the amount of time available, and/or the needs of the patient. If possible, the group member should be allowed to choose the therapist with whom the final interview is to be held. This can be done easily and without self-consciousness by having the group members add their names to a sign-up sheet with different times listed under each therapist's name. In this way patients can choose their preference based on time of day, sex of therapist, therapist style, and familiarity with therapist (e.g., who did the initial screenings, to whom they related most easily during the sessions, etc.).

SESSION 15

Orientation of Group Member to Final Interview

The final interview can be introduced to the group members as follows:

> The purpose of this session is again to assess the progress you've made toward meeting your goals for our group. This should include any areas not mentioned in the last meeting of the group as a whole. Next, we can look at any goals not accomplished and discuss how you may want to make use of the skills you've learned in order to attain them. Following this, we can look to any new goals you may have set recently as well as how to achieve these future goals and/or to cope with these potential stressful situations. Last, I'd very much appreciate any additional feedback you could give me on what the group experience was like for you. It would be very beneficial to future group members if you could tell me what you found most helpful about the group and what could have been more helpful to you. So, our agenda for this session is this:
>
> 1. Review and assessment of goals
> 2. Planning for accomplishment of past remaining goals
> 3. Establishing strategies for new goals
> 4. Preparation for any backsliding in stressful situations
> 5. Feedback on pros and cons of group experience for you
>
> Please feel free to add any additional agenda items for today's session.

Review of Individual Goals and Evaluation of Progress

In preparation for this session, group members were asked to develop a list of areas or problems in their lives which needed additional attention (Appendix 30, part 2). These may include any of the original goals established at the screening session, new problems, and goals recently developed for which the group member believes he needs further preparation.

First, the group member's attention is directed toward the original goals that were developed during the initial group screening session. A more personal and in-depth discussion of which goals were accomplished (Appendix 30, part 1) and specific examples of progress can ensue as a follow-up to work already done in the final group session (Session 14). Patients can disclose additional personal anecdotes that illustrate and reinforce progress made. This exercise also gives the therapist the opportunity to give the patient a thorough assessment, asking questions that can evaluate how well the patient has learned and incorporated the techniques he has been taught. For example, should a patient relate an incident in which he used cognitive restructuring, the therapist could ask "What automatic thought were you able to identify?" and "How were you able to conteract or contradict that thinking?" If the patient has the technique "down pat," the therapist will want to congratulate him on his success. If there is still some misunderstanding or misuse of the technique, the therapist can take this opportunity to reinforce what the patient has learned and to guide him gently in correcting any misconceptions.

Again, just as was done in the preceding group session in front of all the group members, any initial goals not entirely accomplished during the group experience can be addressed.

Formulation of Strategies to Achieve Remaining Goals

The group member is asked to discuss what areas need further effort and what techniques could be used to accomplish the desired ends. Together, the patient and therapist can formulate strategies to deal with the remaining problems. For example, a patient may explain that although he has become increasingly assertive with his wife and is now able to express to her that he needs to have time to be alone, he and his wife are still having difficulty finding mutually enjoyable activities for their time together. Here, the therapist may suggest making use of the problem-solving technique, suggesting that the patient and his wife engage in the problem-solving process as follows: (1) brainstorm a list of potential activities without censoring them; (2) rate and rank each activity in order of mutual acceptability; (3) decide, on the basis of the rank ordering, which activities seem most promising to engage in; and (4) develop tactics to implement the chosen strategy.

Another example is the patient whose daily tension headaches have remitted but who continues to have periodic headaches on particularly stressful occasions. The therapist can examine these occasions with the patient and identify any changes the patient could make in her thinking, her level of muscle tension, or her behavior. Potential strategies could include (1) practicing differential relaxation of the frontalis muscle and sensitizing herself to relax her forehead at the first indication of increased tension; (2) identifying and counteracting the ATs that result in anxiety during problem work situations; (3) evaluating the role increased assertion with co-workers or supervisor could play in decreasing tension in the workplace; and (4) using the problem-solving skills to find solutions to any remaining problems inherent in her particular workplace or work habits.

Developing Future Goals and Planning for Implementation

Often during this group program, patients experience a shift in their goals and expectations for themselves. They frequently move from desiring remission of symptoms to the higher-level goals of self-actualization and the improvement of the quality of their lives. For example, a patient may begin the group with the goal of being able to sleep better, to increase his energy level, and to improve his mood. Once these goals are achieved, this same patient may aspire not only to prevent these symptoms in the future but also to tackle other areas of his life, such as finding a more fulfilling job or making a greater effort to find a mate. Just as the therapist aided the patients in planning strategies for accomplishing goals remaining from the initial list, so too can they work together to plan ways to achieve these new goals.

Therapist Feedback to Patient

During this final session, the therapist can elaborate upon the feedback he gave the group member the previous week, in the last group session. This feedback can include changes the group member has made in his behavior within the group, progress the patient has experienced toward the accomplishment of his articulated goals, and contributions the patient has made to the progress of individual members and the group as a whole.

The following is an example of the type of feedback the therapist could provide:

> You seem a lot more relaxed since the beginning of the group. You've become much more involved with the other group members and also more

willing to talk about yourself. I can tell from your homework, as well as the help you've given others, that you have incorporated the skills of cognitive restructuring and are making good use of them. I was especially impressed with the way you dealt with your automatic thoughts recently, after the misunderstanding you had with your boss. You have obviously become more assertive with her and with your wife as well. Overall, I can see that you've done a lot of hard work in and outside the group and have been a valuable member.

Feedback from the therapist can be more or less congratulatory and more or less extensive than the example above, depending upon the performance of the patient in the group and his self-report of progress.

This part of the session can also include suggestions for future changes. For example:

You've made great strides in limiting the length of your bouts with depression and their severity. To be more successful in warding off depression— that is, in "nipping it in the bud"—you may want to use this depression-free time to develop a compendium of your most typical and most devastating automatic thoughts as well as your best and most convincing rational beliefs. This preparation can be a ready resource when you find yourself becoming upset and can also be used to rehearse reasonable thinking during less stressful times.

The group patients can be encouraged in many different areas to continue to expand upon the growth they've begun during the group experience. For each group member, there are positive changes and behaviors that can be commented upon as well as potential areas for further growth.

The therapist's feedback can be enriched by referring back to the Personal Reminder Forms that the patients fill out after each session. The patient and therapist together can review these forms in discussing accomplishments as well as future goals.

This session is one of the crucial parts of the treatment in that it is the final contact with the group experience for the patient until the six-month booster session, and it can bear heavily upon his overall impression of how well he did in the group and how much he has accomplished.

Patient Feedback to Therapist

This segment of the final session is designed to give the therapist an opportunity to learn more about what was most helpful to the patient about this experience and what could have been improved upon. It also gives the leader another opportunity to learn even more about his style and the patients' reactions to him. Some questions which may help to facilitate this process are as follows:

"What about the group experience did you find particularly beneficial?"

"Which modules did you find most useful and why?"

"What provided the motivation for doing homework outside of the group?"

"Was there any area or skill on which you felt we spent too much time . . . too little time?"

"Was there anything I or my co-leader did that rubbed you the wrong way?"

"How could we improve upon future group programs?"

"Is there any way I or my co-leader could have been more helpful to you?"

The one-to-one atmosphere of this last session should provide useful information that can be noted for future groups. The group members themselves are one of the best sources of suggestions for the improvement of this program; therefore ample time and attention should be allotted for this section of the interview.

Reminder of Six-Month Booster Session

Again, the group member is reminded that there will be a booster session scheduled in six months as a follow-up to the group program. Another card listing the date and time is offered. As was mentioned in the last group session, he is asked to keep a log of problem situations he encounters between this last session and the booster session. For each problem situation, he is asked to list the technique employed to remediate the difficulty and the degree of success attained. (The degree of success is measured in SUD levels; see Session 2). Forms designed for this purpose (see Appendix 31) will be distributed at this time, and the patient is asked to bring the log (or logs) with him to the booster session.

10

BOOSTER SESSIONS — SIX-MONTH FOLLOW-UP SESSION

OVERVIEW

Reorientation
Progress/Accomplishments
Problems That Remain
Homework Assignment

Materials Needed:
1. Individual Goal Sheets
2. Appointment cards with date and time of 12-month follow-up session
3. Log of Problem Situations and Skills Employed (Appendix 31)

BOOSTER SESSION

Introduction

The booster sessions are designed to reinforce and enhance the skill development acquired in the 15-session group sequence. These sessions are also intended to remind the group participant that he is still part of a self-help program—that his public commitment to ongoing growth and the accomplishment of specific goals continues. In addition, the group member may be more willing to become "his own therapist" after only 15 sessions if he is reassured that he can check in again with his group leaders and fellow group members in six months to evaluate how he's doing and receive help as needed for any troublesome areas.

Because brief therapy is a departure from the more traditional longer forms of psychotherapy, patients may tend to feel shortchanged (i.e., that they should remain in treatment until all problem areas are completely resolved). The follow-up groups are helpful in reemphasizing the intent of the coping skills groups (i.e., to present and initiate the practice of skills that will be continuously refined as time goes on). The treatment span is not intended to be limited to the 15 weeks between the first and last sessions.

Reorientation

After six months, some of the group members are likely to have forgotten each other's names. The name game can be resurrected (see Session 1) at this point. Each member is asked to give his first name and an adjective describing himself which begins with the same first letter (or sound) as his first name. He should briefly state why he chose that adjective and, if possible, to recall his original adjective for the sake of comparison. He then repeats the names and accompanying adjectives of each person who preceded him around the group.

Progress/Accomplishments

Each member is asked, in turn, to describe his progress toward his goals as established in the original screening session and in the final session (six months before).

The original goal sheets are distributed as prompts. An example of a patient's six-month report follows:

GROUP MEMBER: I feel really good about reporting that my tension headaches have not returned over the last six months. I practice the relaxation fairly faithfully and am delighted not to be afflicted by those pounding attacks. Except for a bout with the flu in early January. I haven't missed a day of work.

Harvey and I are getting along much better. I don't jump all over him when he's unresponsive or bullheaded. We both seem to have more tolerance for each other. And our daughter, who's mostly away at college, commented on the positive difference in me and us the last time she visited home.

I still find myself getting depressed on occasion, but I catch it much earlier and am able to talk myself out of it. My moods simply don't get the better of me!

Problems That Remain

Following a report from everyone in the group on their achievements, each is called upon in turn to describe those problems that remain. The emphasis is on a solution orientation, where each member is asked to describe his problem, his specific goal for overcoming or dealing with his problems, and what skills might be brought to bear to meet that goal.

An example follows from the same patient who discussed her considerable progress.

GROUP MEMBER: Well, I continue to be a bit of a love addict. I really am overly dependent on Harvey and have a terrible dread of losing him. Mind you, I'm getting better and know that using the homework sheets and the double-column technique on this problem would be very helpful. By the next time we meet, I think I'll be able to report some more rational thinking in that area.

The original sheets are collected and cards listing the time and date of the next booster session are distributed to the group members.

Homework Assignment

Each member is asked to again keep a progress log over the next six months (Appendix 31).

HOMEWORK ASSIGNMENT—SIX-MONTH BOOSTER SESSION

Keep log on progress in meeting goals over next six months.

TWELVE-MONTH BOOSTER SESSION

There is no appreciable difference between the six- and twelve-month booster sessions in terms of their content or the way in which they are conducted. At the conclusion of the second booster session, group members are reminded of the therapists' continued availability, but they are also encouraged to maintain their progress and momentum through concerted application of the skills learned in the coping skills program.

REFERENCES

Authier, J., Gustafson, K., Guerney, B. G., Jr., & Kasdorf, J. A. The psychological practitioner as a teacher: A theoretical, historical and practical review. *Counseling Psychologist*, 1975, 5, 31–50.

Baker, B. L., Kahn, M., & Weiss, J. M. Treatment of insomnia by relaxation. *Journal of Abnormal Psychology*, 1968, 73, 556–558.

Bandura, A. *Principles of behavior modification*. New York: Holt, 1969.

Bandura, A. *Social learning theory*. Englewood Cliffs, N.J.: Prentice-Hall, 1977.

Barrios, B. A., & Shigetomi, C. C. Coping skills training for the management of anxiety: A critical review. *Behavior Therapy*, 1979, 10, 491–522.

Beck, A. T. Thinking and depression. *Archives of General Psychiatry*, 1963, 9, 324–333.

Beck, A. T. *Depression: Clinical, experimental and therapeutic aspects*. New York: Harper & Row, 1967.

Beck, A. T. Cognitive therapy: Nature and relation to behavior therapy. *Behavior Therapy*, 1970. 1, 184–200.

Beck. A. T. Cognition, affect, and psychopathology. *Archives of General Psychiatry*, 1971, 24, 493–500.

Beck, A. T. *Cognitive therapy and the emotional disorders*. New York: International Universities Press, 1976.

Beck, A. T., Rush, A. J., Shaw, B. T., & Emery, G. *Cognitive therapy of depression*. New York: Guilford Press, 1979.

Benson, H. *The relaxation response*. New York: Avon Books, 1975.

Bergin, A. E., & Garfield. S. L. *Handbook of psychotherapy and behavior change: An empirical analysis*. New York: Wiley. 1971.

Bernstein, D. A., & Borkovec, T. D. *Progressive relaxation training: A manual for the helping professions.* Champaign, Ill.: Research Press, 1973.

Bloom, B. S., & Broder, L. J. *Problem-solving processes of college students.* Chicago: University of Chicago Press, 1950.

Brown, S. D. Coping skills training: An evaluation of a psychoeducational program in a community mental health setting. *Journal of Counseling Psychology,* 1980, *27,* 340–345.

Burns. D. D. Personal communication, November 14, 1980. (a)

Burns, D. D. *Feeling good,* New York: Morrow, 1980. (b)

Cautela, J. R. Treatment of compulsive behavior by covert sensitization. *Psychological Record,* 1966, *16,* 33–41.

Cautela, J. R. Covert sensitization. *Psychological Reports,* 1967, *20,* 459–468.

Cautela, J. R. Behavior therapy and self-control: Techniques and implications. In C. M. Franks (Ed.), *Behavior therapy: Appraisal and status.* New York: McGraw-Hill, 1969.

Chambless, D. L., & Goldstein, A. J. Behavioral psychotherapy. In R. J. Corsini (Ed.), *Current Psychotherapies.* Itasca, Ill.: Peacock, 1979.

Cummings, N. A., & Follette, W. T. Psychiatric and medical utilization in a prepaid health plan setting: Part II. *Medical Care,* 1968, *6,* 31–41.

Cummings, N. A., & Follette, W. T. Brief Psychotherapy and Medical Utilization. In H. Dorken & Associates (Eds.), *The professional psychologist today.* San Francisco: Jossey-Bass, 1976.

Cummings, N. A., & VandenBos, G. R. The general practice of psychology. *Professional Psychology,* 1979, *10,* 430–440.

Debus, R. Effects of brief observation of model behavior on conceptual tempo impulsive psychology. *Developmental Psychology,* 1970, *2,* 202–214.

D'Zurilla, T. J., & Goldfried, M. R. Problem solving and behavior modification. *Journal of Abnormal Psychology,* 1971, *78,* 107–126.

Ellis, A. Outcome of employing three techniques of psychotherapy. *Journal of Clinical Psychology,* 1957, *13,* 344–350.

Ellis, A. Rational psychotherapy. *Journal of General Psychology,* 1958, *59,* 35–49.

Ellis, A. *Reason and emotion of psychotherapy.* New York: Lyle Stuart, 1962.

Ellis, A. Rational-emotive therapy in groups. In A. Ellis & R. Grieger (Eds.), *Handbook of rational-emotive therapy.* New York: Springer, 1977.

Ellis, A., & Harper, R. A. *A new guide to rational living.* Englewood Cliffs, N.J.: Prentice-Hall, 1975.

Fleming, B. M., & Thornton, D. W. Coping skills training as a component in the short-term treatment of depression. *Journal of Consulting and Clinical Psychology,* 1980, *48,* 652–654.

Follette, W. T., & Cummings, N. A. Psychiatric services and medical utilization in a prepaid health plan setting. *Medical Care,* 1967, *5,* 25–35.

Galton, F. *Inquiries into human faculty and its development.* London: Macmillan, 1883.

Goldberg, I. D., Krantz, G., & Locke, B. Z. Effect of a short-term outpatient psychiatric therapy benefit on the utilization of medical services in a prepaid group practice medical program. *Medical Care,* 1970, *8,* 419–428.

Goldfried, M. R. The use of relaxation and cognitive relabeling as coping skills. In R. B. Stuart (Ed.), *Behavioral self-management: Strategies, techniques, and outcomes.* New York: Brunner/Mazel, 1977.

Goldfried, M. R., & Davison, G. C. *Clinical behavior therapy.* New York: Holt, 1976.

Goldfried, M. R., & Goldfried, A. P. Cognitive change methods. In E. H. Kanfer & A. P. Goldstein (Eds.), *Helping people change.* New York: Pergamon Press, 1975.

Goldfried, M. R., & Merbaum, M. *Behavior change through self-control.* New York: Holt, 1973.

Goldfried. M. R., & Trier, C. S. Effectiveness of relaxation as an active coping skill. *Journal of Abnormal Psychology,* 1974, *83,* 348–355.

Gordon, T. *Parent effectiveness training.* New York: Peter H. Wyden, 1970.

Guerney, B. G., Jr., Stollack, G., & Guerney, L. A format for a new mode of psychological practice: Or how to escape a zombie. *Counseling Psychologist,* 1970, *2,* 97–104.

Guerney, B. G., Jr., Stollack, G., & Guerney, L. Practicing psychologist as educator: An alternative to the medical practitioner model. *Professional Psychology,* 1971, *2,* 276–282.

Harlow, H. F. The formation of learning sets. *Psychological Review,* 1949. *56,* 51–65.

Heidl, F. J., & Borkovec, T. D. Relaxation-induced anxiety: Paradoxical anxiety enhancement due to relaxation training, *Journal of Consulting and Clinical Psychology,* 1983, *51,* 171–182.

Hilgard, E. R., Atkinson, R. C., & Atkinson, R. L. *Introduction to psychology (6th ed.).* New York, Harcourt Brace Jovanovich, 1975.

Jacobson, E. *Progressive relaxation (2nd ed.).* Chicago: University of Chicago Press, 1938.

Jakubowski-Spector, P. Facilitating the growth of women through assertive training. *The Counseling Psychologist,* 1973, *4,* 75–86.

Janis, I. Psychodynamic aspects of stress tolerance. In S. Klausner (Ed.). *The quest for self-control.* New York: Free Press, 1965.

Jeffrey R. W., Gerber, W. M., Rosenthal, B. S. & Lindquist, R. A. Monetary contracts in weight control: Effectiveness of group and individual contracts of varying size. *Journal of Consulting and Clinical Psychology,* 1983, *51,* 242–248.

Kanfer, F. H. The many faces of self-control or behavior modification changes its focus. In R. B. Stuart (Ed.). *Behavioral self-management.* New York: Brunner/Mazel, 1977.

Kanfer, F. H., & Goldstein, A. P. *Helping people change: A textbook of methods.* New York: Pergamon Press, 1975.

Kanfer, F. H., & Phillips, J. S. *Learning foundations of behavior therapy.* New York: Wiley, 1970.

Krumboltz, J., & Thoreson, C. *Behavioral counseling: Cases and techniques.* New York: Holt, 1969.

Lange, H., & Jakubowski. P. *Responsible assertive behavior: Cognitive-behavioral procedures for trainers.* Champaign, Ill.: Research Press, 1976.

Lazarus, A. A. New methods in psychotherapy: A case study. *South African Medical Journal*, 1958, *33*, 660.

Lazarus, A. A. Behavior therapy in groups. In G. M. Gazda (Ed.), *Basic approaches to group psychotherapy and group counseling*. Springfield, Ill.: Charles C Thomas, 1968.

Lazarus, A. A. *Behavior therapy and beyond*. New York: McGraw-Hill, 1971.

Lieberman, M. A., Yalom, I. D., & Miles. M. B. *Encounter groups, First facts*. New York: Basic Books, 1973.

Lindsley, O. R., & Skinner, B. F. A method for the experimental analysis of the behavior of psychotic patients. *American Psychologist*, 1954, *9*, 419–420.

Mahoney, M. J. *Cognition and behavior modification*. Cambridge, Mass.: Ballinger, 1974.

Mahoney, M. J. Personal science: A cognitive learning therapy. In A. Ellis & R. Grieger (Eds.), *Handbook of rational psychotherapy*. New York: Springer, 1977.

Mahoney, M. J., & Thoresen, C. E. *Self-control: Power to the person*. Monterey, Calif.: Brooks Cole, 1974.

McDougall, W. *Outline of psychology*. New York: Scribner's, 1923.

Meichenbaum, D. H. Cognitive modification of test-anxious college students. *Journal of Consulting and Clinical Psychology*, 1972, *39*, 370–380.

Meichenbaum, D. H. A self-instructional approach to stress management: A proposal for stress inoculation training. In C. D. Spielberger & I. G. Sarason (Eds.), *Stress and anxiety*. New York: Wiley, 1973.

Meichenbaum, D. H. Self-instructional methods. In F. H. Kanfer & A. P. Goldstein (Eds.), *Helping people change*. New York: Pergamon Press, 1975.

Meichenbaum, D. H. *Cognitive-behavior modification: An integrative approach*. New York: Plenum Press, 1977.

Meichenbaum, D. H., Gilmore, B., & Fedoravicius, A. Group insight versus group desensitization in treating speech anxiety. *Journal of Consulting and Clinical Psychology*, 1971, *36*. 410–421.

Meichenbaum, D. H., Turk, D., & Bernstein, S. The nature of coping with stress. In I. Sarason & C. Spielberger (Eds.), *Stress and anxiety* (Vol. 2). New York: Wiley, 1975.

Miller, G. A. Psychology as a means of promoting human welfare. *American Psychologist*. 1969, *24*, 1063–1075.

Murphy, L. *The widening world of childhood*. New York: Basic Books, 1962.

Patterson, G. R. Reprogramming the families of aggressive boys. In C. E. Thoresen (Ed.), *Behavior modification in education*. Chicago: University of Chicago Press. 1973.

Rogers, C. R. *Client-centered therapy*. Boston: Houghton Mifflin, 1951.

Seligman, M. *Helplessness: On depression, development and death*. San Francisco: Freeman, 1975.

Shaffer, C. S., Shapiro, J., Sank, L. I., & Coghlan, D. J. Positive changes in depression, anxiety and assertion following individual and group cognitive behavior therapy intervention. *Cognitive Therapy and Research*, 1981, *5*, 149–157.

Shaffer, C. S.. Sank, L. I., Shapiro, J., & Donovan, D. C. Group versus individual cognitive behavior therapy: Six-month follow-up. *Journal of Group Therapy, Psychodrama, and Sociometry*, 1982, *35*(2), 57–64.

Shapiro, J., Sank, L. I., Shaffer, C. S., & Donovan. D. C. Cost effectiveness of individual versus group cognitive behavior therapy for problems of depression and anxiety in an HMO population. *Journal of Clinical Psychology*, 1982, *38*(3), 674–677.

Shapiro, J. R., Shaffer, C. S., Sank, L. I., & Coghlan, D. J. Cognitive behavior therapy groups: Methods and comparative research. In D. Upper & S. M. Ross (Eds.), *Behavior group therapy*. Champaign, Ill.: Research Press, 1981.

Sherman, A. R. Real-life exposure as a primary therapeutic factor in the desensitization treatment of fear. *Journal of Abnormal Psychology*, 1972, *79*, 19–28.

Skinner, B. F. *Science and human behavior*. New York, Macmillan, 1953.

Smith, M. J. *When I say no I feel guilty*. New York: Dial Press, 1975.

Steinmetz. J. L., Antonuccio, D., & Lewinsohn. P. M. *Prediction of individual outcome in a group intervention for depression*. Unpublished manuscript, V. A. Medical Center, Palo Alto, Calif., 1981.

Suinn, R. M., & Richardson, F. Anxiety management training: A nonspecific behavior therapy program for anxiety control. *Behavior Therapy*, 1971, *2*, 498–510.

Thoresen, C. E., & Mahoney, M. J. *Behavioral self-control*. New York: Holt, 1974.

Upper, D., & Ross, S. M. *Behavioral group therapy, 1980: An annual review*. Champaign, Ill.: Research Press, 1980.

Weiss, R. S. The emotional impact of marital separation. *Journal of Social Issues*, 1976, *32*(1), 135–145.

Wolpe, J. *Psychotherapy by reciprocal inhibition*. Stanford, Calif.: Stanford University Press, 1958.

Wolpe, J., & Lazarus, A. A. *Behavior therapy techniques*. New York: Pergamon Press, 1966.

Wolpin, M.. & Raines, J. Visual imagery, expected roles and extinction as possible factors in reducing fear and avoidance behavior. *Behavior Research and Therapy*, 1966, *4*, 25–37.

Yalom, I. D. *The theory and practice of group psychotherapy*. New York: Basic Books, 1970.

Zeiss, A. M., Lewinsohn, P. M., & Munoz, R. F. Non-specific improvement effects in depression using interpersonal skills training, pleasant activities schedules or cognitive training. *Journal of Consulting and Clinical Psychology*, 1979, *47*, 427–439.

PRETREATMENT QUESTIONNAIRE (PTQ)

Name _____ Date _____

Address _____ Zip _____

Work phone _____ Home phone _____

Age _____ Occupation _____

Now employed? Yes ( ) No ( ) Position _____

Name of organization _____ Where? _____

Last grade of school completed _____

IN CASE OF EMERGENCY, PLEASE NOTIFY _____

Relationship _____ Home phone _____ Work phone _____

With whom do you live?   (e.g., parents, spouse, roommate, friend)

_____

Who referred you? _____

Please indicate your marital status (circle one):

Engaged   Remarried   Divorced   Separated   Widowed   Single   Married

I. Presenting Problem

A. Briefly state the nature of your problem(s):

_____

_____

_____

_____

_____

B. Please indicate briefly how your present problems developed over time:

_____

_____

_____

_____

_____

_____

C. How severe is your most pressing problem? Please rate from 1 to 7:

   1   2   3   4   5   6   7

   Slightly   Almost   Incapacitating

   upsetting   overwhelming

D. Have you ever seen anyone for a psychological problem?

   Yes ( ) No ( ) Whom? _____

   Where? (facility and city) _____

   When? _____ Circumstances _____

E. Have you seen anyone for this current problem?

   Yes ( ) No ( ) Whom? _____

   Where? (facility and city) _____

   When? _____

F. Have you ever been hospitalized for a psychological problem?

   Yes ( ) No ( ) If yes, name of hospital _____

   _____ City and state _____

   Dates of hospitalization _____ Diagnosis _____

   _____ Circumstances _____

If he or she deems necessary, does your therapist have permission to contact your past therapist(s) or facility(ies) to obtain your past records?

Yes ( ) No ( ) If yes, please sign below.

_____   _____

Signature   Date

G. Have you ever seriously considered taking your own life?

   Yes ( ) No ( ) If yes, when? _____

   Do you feel this way now? _____

   Have you ever attempted to take your own life? _____

   If yes, how and when? _____

   _____

H. When was your last medical examination? _____

   Name of practitioner _____

   Please list all medications you are currently taking including over-the-counter medicines (birth control, etc.).

_____

_____

Please list your major health problems. _____

_____

J. Please list your three principal fears:

   (1) _____

   (2) _____

   (3) _____

K. Please list hobbies, activities, and other interests:

_____

_____

    L. How do you spend most of your free time?

_____

_____

    M. Do you tend to make friends easily? _____

       Once you have made friends, do you keep them? _____

II. Vocational Information

    A. How are you employed at present? _____

    B. What kinds of positions have you held in the past?

_____

_____

    C. Have you ever been fired from a job? Yes ( ) No ( ) If yes, briefly describe
       circumstances. _____

_____

    D. Are you satisfied with your present job? Yes ( ) No ( )
       If not, please indicate the ways in which you are dissatisfied:

_____

_____

    E. What is your present income? _____
       Do your expenses exceed your income? Yes ( ) No ( )
       If yes, by how much? _____

    F. Goals:
       What were your goals in the past? _____
       What are your goals now? _____

_____

_____

    G. Military Service:
       Are your currently or have you ever served in the armed forces?
       Yes ( ) No ( )
       If yes, branch _____
       Rank _____ Discharge (e.g., honorable) _____

    H. Legal Problems:
       Have you ever been tried in a court of law for other than a minor traffic violation?
       Yes ( ) No ( )
       If yes, please detail. _____

_____

       Have you ever been imprisoned? Yes ( ) No ( )
       If yes, please detail. _____

_____

III. Sexual History

    A. What were the attitudes of your parents towards your sexuality and what was
       the extent of sexual instruction in your home?

_____

_____

B. When and how did you first learn about sex? _____

_____

C. Are you satisfied with your present sex life? Yes (   ) No (   )
   If not, in what ways could it be improved?

_____

_____

D. Males:
   Do you currently or have you ever had erectile problems?

_____

   Do you currently or have you ever had problems having an orgasm too quickly or
   not at all? Yes (   ) No (   ) If yes, please explain.

_____

E. Females:
   Do you currently have or have you ever had problems becoming aroused?

_____

   Do you find intercourse painful? _____

   Do you currently or have you ever had problems reaching orgasm? _____

_____

   Do you have any menstrual problems? _____

_____

   Do your periods affect your moods? _____

_____

F. Is there anything else that your therapist should know about your first or any
   subsequent sexual experience? Yes (   ) No (   )
   If yes, please explain. _____

_____

_____

IV. Relationships

   A. Marital Information (If never married, start with Part B)
      How long have you been married? _____
      How long did you know your spouse before you were engaged?_____
      How long did you know your spouse before you were married? _____
      Spouse's name _____ Spouse's age _____
      Spouse's education _____
      Spouse's occupation _____
      Briefly describe your spouse's personality. _____

_____

      In what areas are you and your spouse most compatible?

_____

_____

In what areas are you and your spouse least compatible?

_____

_____

Are there any problems in your relationship with your in-laws?
Yes ( ) No ( ) If yes, please describe.

_____

Have you been married before? Yes ( ) No ( ) If yes, please give any relevant details.

_____

_____

Have you or your spouse had any miscarriages or abortions? Yes ( ) No ( ) If yes, please give any relevant details.

_____

_____

B. Other Relationships

Are you at present romantically involved with one individual?
Yes ( ) No ( ) If yes, for how long? _____

Partner's name _____ Partner's age _____

Partner's education _____

Partner's occupation _____

Briefly describe your partner's personality. _____

In what areas are you and your partner most compatible?

_____

In what areas are you and your partner least compatible?

_____

Have you or your partner had any miscarriages or abortions? Yes ( ) No ( )
If yes, please give any relevant details. _____

_____

C. Children

How many children do you have? _____

Please list the name, sex, and age of each child (include stepchildren). _____

_____

_____

Do any of your children present special problems? Yes ( ) No ( )
If yes, please explain. _____

_____

D. Social Relationships

Describe the positive aspects of your present social life. _____

_____

_____

Describe any difficulties/shortcomings that you experience in your current social relationships. _____

_____

_____

Briefly add any information about prior relationships which you feel may be important in understanding any current problems. _____

_____

_____

V. Familial Information

A. Father:

Is your father living? Yes ( ) No ( )

If he is deceased, how old were you at the time of his death? _____

Cause of death _____ Age at death _____

If your father is alive, what is his present age? _____

What was the last grade of school that he completed? _____

What is his occupation? _____

How is his current health? _____

Briefly describe your father's personality. Please describe your relationship with him in the past as well as currently.

_____

_____

_____

B. Mother:

Is your mother living? Yes ( ) No ( )

If she is deceased, how old were you at the time of her death? _____

Cause of death _____ Age at death _____

If your mother is alive, what is her present age? _____

What was the last grade of school that she completed? _____

What is her occupation? _____

How is her current health? _____

Briefly describe your mother's personality. Please describe your relationship with her in the past as well as currently.

_____

_____

_____

C. Siblings:

Please list names and ages of brothers/sisters—indicate if step (S) or half (H):

Brothers   Sisters

_____   _____

_____   _____

Please describe your relationship with your brothers/sisters:

Past: _____

_____

_____

Present: _____
_____
_____

D. Childhood:
In what ways did your parents or guardians punish you as a child?
_____

Please describe the atmosphere of the home in which you grew up, including your parents' relationship with each other.
_____
_____
_____

Were you able to share confidences with your parents?
_____

If you were raised by someone other than your parents, who did raise you and during what period?
_____

If you have a stepparent, how old were you when your parent remarried? _____
Sex of stepparent _____ Please describe your relationship with your step-parent. _____
_____
_____

Within what religion were you brought up? _____
_____

Briefly describe any religious training you received:
_____
_____

E. Adulthood:
What is your current religious affiliation? _____
What role does religion play in your current life?
_____

Have your parents, relatives, or friends ever significantly interfered in your personal life, marriage, occupation, etc.? Yes ( ) No ( ) If yes, please describe:
_____
_____

Who in your life would you currently identify as being most important? (You may list several.) _____
_____

F. Medical/Psychological Background:
Does any member of your family suffer from alcohol/drug problems? Please give details: _____
_____
_____

Does any member of your family suffer from any mental, emotional, or nervous disorder? Yes (   ) No (   ) Please give details:

_____

_____

Does any member of your family suffer from any other illnesses which might be relevant? Please give details:

_____

_____

Do you have any past or current medical problems that are a source of concern to you? Yes (   ) No (   ) Please give details:

_____

_____

VI. Please indicate which of the following are current problems for you by drawing a line under the items that apply. For example, if feeling tense is a problem for you, you would draw a line under the word Tense.

A. Mood Problems
   001. Depressed
   002. Tense
   003. Unable to relax
   004. Panicky
   005. Too nervous or high-strung
   006. Easily upset
   007. Irritable or easily angered
   008. Lonely
   009. Easily hurt, too sensitive
   010. Constantly worried
   011. Crying more frequently
   012. Without pleasure in life
   013. Losing interest in things in general
   014. Thinking about ending my life
   015. Wishing I were dead
   016. Anxious
   017. Hopeless
   018. Crying uncontrollably
   019. Bitter
   020. Sad or blue
   021. Discontented
   022. Lost or adrift
   023. Guilty
   024. Easily bored

B. Cognitive Problems
   025. Having difficulty remembering recent events
   026. Having difficulty remembering things in the past
   027. Confused
   028. Disoriented

O29. Having concentration difficulties
O30. Having trouble understanding what I read
O31. Inefficient in work and study
O32. Daydreaming
O33. Having difficulty thinking clearly
O34. Hearing voices
O35. Seeing visions
O36. Having strange or unreal feelings

C. Work and Financial Concerns
O37. Unable to make a vocational choice
O38. Unable to enter chosen vocation
O39. Dissatisfied with my vocational choice
O40. Difficulty in combining marriage and career
O41. Working too hard
O42. Not interested or challenged at work
O43. Receiving little recognition for work done
O44. Not satisfied with working conditions
O45. Afraid of losing my job
O46. Having problems with co-workers or supervisors
O47. Financial difficulties
O48. Unable to handle responsibility
O49. Not getting to work on time or leaving too early

D. Social and Family Concerns
O50. Having difficulty making friends
O51. Feeling uncomfortable with other people
O52. Having too few dates
O53. Not finding a suitable life partner
O54. Having difficulty deciding whether to get married or making a long-term commitment
O55. Having to break up a love affair
O56. Caring for more than one person
O57. Frequent arguments with spouse or partner
O58. Having different interests from spouse or partner
O59. Breaking up my marriage/relationship
O60. Difficulty in deciding whether to have children
O61. Having problems with child-rearing
O62. Feeling rejected by family
O63. Poor relationship with mother/father (circle one or both)
O64. Having difficulty with roommate(s)
O65. Unhappy where I am living
O66. Not managing regular chores
O67. Withdrawing from other people
O68. Feeling rejected by friends
O69. Feeling rejected by a loved one
O70. Not in love with spouse or partner (circle one)

E. Sexual Concerns
   071. Lacking information about sex
   072. Finding it difficult to control sexual impulses
   073. Bothered by sexual thoughts or dreams
   074. Worried about effects of masturbation
   075. Sexually attracted to someone of the same sex
   076. Sexually unsatisfied
   077. Experiencing sexual desires different from partner(s)
   078. Repelled by thoughts of sexual relations
   079. Experiencing erectile difficulties
   080. Premature ejaculation
   081. Having difficulty becoming sexually aroused
   082. Having difficulty in reaching orgasm
   083. Finding intercourse painful or impossible (circle one)
   084. Worried about pregnancy
   085. Losing interest in sex
   086. Unwanted sexual thoughts or desires

F. Somatic Concerns
   087. Headaches
   088. Rapid heartbeat or chest pains (circle one)
   089. Bowel disturbances
   090. Too little or too much sleep (circle one)
   091. Dizziness
   092. Stomach trouble
   093. Fatigue
   094. Fainting spells
   095. Poor appetite or overeating (circle one)
   096. Tremors
   097. Anxiety attacks
   098. Poor complexion or skin problems
   099. Muscular aches and pains
   100. Hypertension (high blood pressure)
   101. Too much overweight or underweight (circle one)
   102. Alcohol problems
   103. Drug-related problems
   104. Smoking
   105. Hyperventilation (rapid breathing)
   106. Muscle weakness or fatigue
   107. Menstrual problems (including pain)
   108. Recent weight loss
   109. Recent weight gain
   110. Excessive pain
   111. Other medical problems (that I worry about) _____

G. Feelings about Oneself
   112. Lacking self-confidence

113. Lacking leadership ability
114. Not being smart enough
115. Timid or shy (nonassertive)
116. Taking things too seriously
117. Too short or too tall (circle one)
118. Physically unattractive
119. Lacking ambition
120. Too easily influenced by others
121. Too careless
122. Not able to do anything well
123. Too self-centered
124. Feeling worthless
125. Feeling guilty
126. Feeling helpless
127. Blame myself for things
128. Feeling misunderstood
129. Feeling unloved
130. Feeling restless
131. Unable to make decisions
132. Feeling ashamed of something
133. Feeling things are out of control
134. Not flexible enough

H. Value and Religious Concerns
135. Needing a philosophy of life
136. Not knowing the kind of person I want to be
137. Confused as to what I really want
138. Feeling life is not worthwhile
139. Confused in religious beliefs
140. Losing earlier religious beliefs
141. Not getting satisfactory answers from religion

I. Behavior Problems
142. Unable to control certain repetitive behavior
143. Engaged in unlawful or dangerous behavior (circle one)
144. Having bad or dangerous personal habits
145. Smoking excessively
146. Biting nails or cuticles
147. Pulling or chewing hair (circle one)
148. Drinking excessively
149. Using drugs excessively
150. Taking unnecessary risks
151. Driving unsafely
152. Gambling excessively
153. Unable to slow down
154. Unable to act rapidly
155. Having temper tantrums

156. Being quarrelsome
157. Having unwanted sexual habits

J. Other Problems (please specify)
158. _____
159. _____
160. _____

Please look back over the items you have underlined and *circle* the number in front of the problems you would like to deal with in therapy. For example, if you have difficulty making friends and would like to deal with this in therapy, you would circle the number (050) in front of the underlined words Having difficulty making friends.

What are the *three* most disturbing problems for you at this time? Please designate their numbers: _____

Do you feel that this gives an accurate picture of your problems? _____

If not, please comment _____

_____

VII. Additional Information

A. Please describe any upsetting or traumatic experiences not mentioned earlier in this questionnaire:

_____
_____
_____

B. Please describe those situations in which you feel most anxious:

_____
_____
_____

C. Please describe those situations in which you feel most relaxed:

_____
_____
_____

D. Have you ever been in a situation in which you have felt out of control?
Yes (   ) No (   ) Please describe:

_____
_____

E. What goals would you hope to attain from a psychotherapy experience?

_____
_____
_____

F. Please add any other pertinent information not previously covered that might assist your therapist in your treatment and/or evaluation:

_____
_____
_____
_____

APPENDIX 2

PREGROUP SCREENING DESCRIPTION OF THE COPING SKILLS GROUP

You have been referred to the Coping Skills Group by your therapist. The following is a description of the four modules that constitute this group experience. After each description, you will find a group of problem areas that can be alleviated or lessened by the skills taught in that particular module. As you read each description, please think about yourself and why you are seeking assistance. You will then meet for 20 minutes with one of the group leaders, who will aid you in developing personal goals for your group experience. We hope that by participating in this pregroup goal-setting session your benefit from the group sessions will be maximized.

THE RELAXATION MODULE

The first module exposes the participant to two different relaxation procedures—Deep Muscle Relaxation (DMR) and Benson's Relaxation Response (BRR). Both techniques teach a skill that counters bodily experiences of stress and psychological experiences of anxiety. Group members with somatic problems such as chronic lower back pain, tension headaches, problems of reduced efficiency at work, or anxiety in social circumstances are especially likely to benefit from these techniques. However, *most* people are at some point inappropriately tense and can benefit from the mastery of these skills.

Examples of Problem Areas:
1. Difficulty falling asleep
2. Persistent tension headaches
3. Feeling "tied up in knots" on the job

THE COGNITIVE RESTRUCTURING MODULE

This module is based on the theory that extreme negative emotions are not the result of life experiences but rather of the attitudes or thoughts one has about these experiences. Cognitive restructuring is a skill that involves recognizing unreasonable thoughts, challenging these thoughts, and developing more appropriate and rational sentences to say to oneself. This more rational thinking eventuates in the lessening and/or prevention of excessive emotional states such as severe depression and anxiety, extreme anger, and exaggerated jealousy.

Examples of Problem Areas:
1. Sleeplessness
2. Loss of appetite
3. Depressed mood
4. Anxious mood
5. Loss of interest in things
6. Concentration difficulties

THE ASSERTION-TRAINING MODULE

This module will seek to teach assertion skills. Assertion is the ability to make one's needs known without doing so at the expense of other people. Group members with difficulties in standing up for themselves, making requests of others, or turning down unreasonable requests from others will find this section especially helpful. Role playing and homework assignments ready the group member to meet the specific goals that each is expected to state at the beginning of the module.

Examples of Problem Areas:
1. Expressing positive feelings to a loved one
2. Turning down a neighbor's request to borrow a favorite, fragile object
3. Saying no to a boss's demand for overtime work

THE PROBLEM-SOLVING MODULE

This fourth and last module is devoted to teaching a strategy for solving life problems. A step-by-step approach is emphasized; it is adaptable to the full range of problems with which the group member might be confronted in the work, social, or familial environment. Group members who feel weighed down or overwhelmed by problem situations will find this module especially useful. They will be given an opportunity to discuss this approach's applicability to the problems which they specify at the outset of the module.

Examples of Problem Areas:
1. Finding a satisfactory job
2. Finding a mate
3. Living within one's financial means

LIST OF SYMPTOMS COMMON TO PATIENTS REFERRED TO THE COPING SKILLS GROUP

1. Symptoms of depression
    a. Sleep deprivation
    b. Loss of appetite
    c. Dysphoria
    d. Decreased libido
    e. Concentration difficulties
    f. Fatigue

2. Symptoms of anxiety
    a. Increased muscle tension
    b. Headaches
    c. Gastrointestinal problems
    d. Irritability
    e. Heart palpitations
    f. Sweating
    g. Hyperventilation

3. Problems of assertion
    a. Difficulty in expressing feelings
    b. Difficulty in responding to criticism
    c. Inability to assert oneself with loved ones
    d. Problem in asserting oneself with strangers

4. Problems in living
    a. Inability to find a satisfying job

b. Difficulty finding an "eligible" date
c. Problems in "making ends meet" (i.e., financial difficulties)
d. Difficulties meeting an "overwhelming" work or school assignment

APPENDIX 4

POTENTIAL GOALS FOR EACH MODULE

A. Relaxation Module
   1. Be able to fall asleep faster
   2. Be able to fall back to sleep easily after awakening in the middle of the night
   3. Relieve the pain in my (lower) back
   4. Reduce the frequency of my tension headaches
   5. Not feel so tied up in knots at the end of my work day

B. Cognitive Restructuring Module
   1. Feel more in control of negative mood states
      a. Avoid becoming inappropriately angry
      b. Decrease tendency to become "unavoidably" depressed
      c. Experience fewer negative changes in energy level, sexual interest, appetite, sleep patterns, sociability, sense of humor
   2. Increase efficiency at work, decrease distractability
   3. Feel more in control in important (romantic, career, social) relationships

C. Assertion-Training Module
   1. Be able to say no to unreasonable requests from my co-workers
   2. Be able to tell my partner about things that bother me without blaming
   3. Be able to accept compliments without becoming embarrassed or denying their validity
   4. Be able to show interest in someone and initiate social contact

D. Problem-Solving Module
   1. Find a job that is more satisfying but as lucrative as the one I hold presently

2. Meet more people and increase my social activities
3. Increase the amount of free time I have available to me in order to pursue more of my interests

COPING SKILLS GROUP SCREENING FORM – INDIVIDUAL GOAL SHEET

GOALS FOR TREATMENT*

I. Relaxation Module

    a. _____

       _____

    b. _____

       _____

    c. _____

       _____

II. Cognitive Restructuring Module

    a. _____

       _____

    b. _____

       _____

    c. _____

       _____

III. Assertion-Training Module

    a. _____

       _____

    b. _____

       _____

*To be filled out by screening therapist.

c. _____
   _____

IV. Problem-Solving Module
   a. _____
      _____
   b. _____
      _____
   c. _____
      _____

COPING SKILLS GROUP ATTENDANCE/ PERFORMANCE RECORD AND CONTRACT

NAME _____   DATE _____

Session	1	2	3	4	5	6	7	8	9	10	11	12	13	14	15
Dates															
Attendance															
Punctuality															
Written Homework															
Readings															
Buddy Contact															
Deposit Remaining															

Key		Amount Deducted	
PA	= Planned absence	Nonattendance	$10
+	= Accomplished	Nonattendance with call	$ 5
O	= Not accomplished	Incomplete written homework	$ 2
O/C	= Absent but called	Incomplete reading	$ 2
O/C	= Late but called	No buddy contact	$ 2
N/A	= Not applicable	Lateness	$ 2
		Lateness with call	$ 1
		Planned absence	$ 0

In an effort to maximize the learning of effective coping skills, a voluntary refundable deposit of $20 is requested of each coping skills group participant. This deposit is not required and participation in the program is not contingent upon the posting of this deposit. (However, compliance with the requirements of attendance, punctuality, buddy contact, and completion of reading and written assignments is mandatory for all members.)

I understand that the deposit is nonmandaory and agree to the conditions for the return of my deposit and the schedule of penalties for noncompliance.

Signature _____ Date _____

APPENDIX 7

EXAMPLE OF COMPLETED COPING SKILLS GROUP SCREENING FORM — INDIVIDUAL GOAL SHEET

GOALS FOR TREATMENT*

I. Relaxation Module
   a. I want to eliminate my tension headaches.
   b. I want to fall asleep more quickly on weekday nights.
   c. _____

II. Cognitive-Restructuring Module
   a. I want to get less angry at my spouse when he drinks too much at parties.
   b. I want to feel less depressed about my sex life.
   c. I want to be less jealous of my spouse's career advances.

III. Assertion-Training Module
   a. I want to ask my boss for my overdue promotion.
   b. I want my children to help me with meal preparation.
   c. _____

IV. Problem-Solving Module
   a. I want to make more friends.
   b. I want to advance my career.
   c. I want my spouse to join an alcoholism rehabilitation program.

*To be filled out by screening therapist

209

APPENDIX 8

RELAXATION PRACTICE LOG

Name

Day	Date	RR* + = yes O = no	Sessions Twice daily	Time Begun	Time Ended	Beginning SUD level	Ending SUD level	Scenes used C = competency P = pleasant	Comments (e.g., distracting or enhancing variables)
1			S1 DMR**						
			S2 DMR						
2			S1 DMR						
			S2 DMR						
3			S1 DMR						
			S2 DMR						

Continued

Day	Date	RR* + = yes O = no	Sessions Twice daily	Time Begun	Time Ended	Beginning SUD level	Ending SUD level	Scenes used C = competency P = pleasant	Comments (e.g., distracting or enhancing variables)
4			S1 DMR						
			S2 DMR						
5			S1 DMR						
			S2 DMR						
6			S1 DMR						
			S2 DMR						
7			S1 DMR						
			S2 DMR						

*RR = Relaxation Response.
**DMR = Deep Muscle Relaxation.

LIST OF REQUIRED AND SUGGESTED READINGS

REQUIRED READINGS

1. Burns, D. D. *Feeling good.* New York: Morrow, 1980.
2. Smith, M. J. *When I say no I feel guilty.* New York: Bantam, 1975.

SUGGESTED READINGS

1. Ellis, A., Harper, R. A. *A new guide to rational living.* Englewood Cliffs, N. J.: Prentice-Hall, 1975. (Also in paperback. North Hollywood, California: Wilshire Books, 1975)
2. Benson, H. *The relaxation response.* New York: Avon, 1975.
3. Dyer, W. *Your Erroneous Zones.* New York: Avon, 1977.

APPENDIX 10

PERSONAL REMINDER FORM

Session _____ Module _____ Date _____

I. What I got out of this session:
    A. Skills
        1. _____
        2. _____
        3. _____
    B. Insights
        1. _____
        2. _____
        3. _____
II. What I intend to work on for next session:
    A. Intrapersonal (involving myself only)
        1. _____
        2. _____
        3. _____
    B. Interpersonal
        1. _____
        2. _____
        3. _____

APPENDIX 11

EXAMPLE OF COMPLETED PERSONAL REMINDER FORM

Session <u>4</u>   Module <u>Cognitive restructuring</u>   Date <u>May 19, 1983</u>

I. What I got out of this session:

  A. Skills

    1. <u>Knowing what an AT is.</u>

    2. <u>How to use a "dispute handle."</u>

    3. _____

  B. Insights

    1. <u>Sometimes I'll find myself thinking like I'm depressed and be using distorted thinking.</u>

    2. _____

    3. _____

II. What I intend to work on for next session:

  A. Intrapersonal (involving myself only)

    1. <u>Try to catch myself in distorted thinking some more.</u>

    2. _____

    3. _____

  B. Interpersonal

    1. <u>Talk to my girlfriend about when she sees me using ATs.</u>

    2. _____

    3. _____

APPENDIX 12

RELAXATION SEQUENCE

BODY PART	CUE
Fingers and hands	Clench
Wrists and forearms	Bend back
Biceps	Strong-man act
Triceps	Sleepwalker — elbows locked
Shoulders	Hunch
Forehead	Raise eyebrows, frown
Eyes	Squint
Lips	Purse, suck on a lemon
Jaw	Jutting lower jaw outward
Tongue	Roof of mouth
Throat	Yawn, say "ahh"
Neck	Rotate — left, right, back, forward
Chest cavity	Deep breath, slow exhalation
Chest and upper back	Shoulders back, chest pushed out
Abdomen	Push out stomach, pull all the way in
Lower back	Arched
Buttocks	Clenched
Thighs and legs — I	Knees locked, feet pointed up
Thighs and legs — II	Knees locked, feet pointed down
Toes and feet — I	Toes curled down
Toes and feet — II	Toes curled upward

APPENDIX 13

COGNITIVE DISTORTIONS

1. **All-or-Nothing Thinking:** You see things in black and white categories. If your performance falls short of perfect, you see yourself as a total failure.
2. **Overgeneralization:** You see a single negative event as a never-ending pattern.
3. **Mental Filter:** You pick out a single negative detail and dwell on it exclusively, so that your vision of all reality becomes darkened, like the drop of ink that discolors the entire beaker of water.
4. **Disqualifying the Positive:** You reject positive experiences by insisting they "don't count" for some reason or other. In this way you can maintain a negative belief that is contradicted by your everyday experiences.
5. **Jumping to Conclusions:** You make a negative interpretation even though there are no definite facts that convincingly support your conclusion.

   a. **Mind Reading.** You arbitrarily conclude that someone is reacting negatively to you, and you don't bother to check this out.
   b. **The Fortune-Teller Error.** You anticipate that things will turn out badly, and you feel convinced that your prediction is an already established fact.

From "You Feel the Way You Think" in *Feeling Good: The New Mood Therapy* by David D. Burns. New York: William Morrow, 1980; Signet Edition, 1981. Copyright © 1980 by David D. Burns. Reprinted by permission of the author and the publisher.

6. **Magnification (Catastrophizing) or Minimization:** You exaggerate the importance of things (such as your goof-up or someone else's achievement), or you inappropriately shrink things until they appear tiny (your own desirable qualities or the other fellow's imperfections). This is also called the "binocular trick."

7. **Emotional Reasoning:** You assume that your negative emotions necessarily reflect the way things really are: "I feel it, therefore it must be true."

8. **"Should" Statements:** You try to motivate yourself with "shoulds" and "shouldn'ts," as if you had to be whipped and punished before you could be expected to do anything. "Musts" and "oughts" are also offenders. The emotional consequence is guilt. When you direct "should" statements toward others, you feel anger, frustration, and resentment.

9. **Labeling and Mislabeling:** This is an extreme form of overgeneralization. Instead of describing your error, you attach a negative label to yourself: "I'm a loser." When someone else's behavior rubs you the wrong way, you attach a negative label onto him: "He's a goddam louse." Mislabeling involves describing an event with language that is highly colored and emotionally loaded.

10. **Personalization:** You see yourself as the cause of some negative external event for which, in fact, you were not primarily responsible.

APPENDIX 14

DISPUTE HANDLES

Do I know for certain that _____ will happen?

Am I 100 percent sure of these awful consequences?

What evidence do I have that _____?

Does _____ have to equal or lead to _____?

Do I have a crystal ball?

What is the worst that could happen? How bad is that?

Could there be any other explanations?

What is the likelihood that _____?

Is _____ really so important or consequential?

Does _____'s opinion reflect that of everyone else?

Is _____ really so important that my entire future resides with its outcome?

HOMEWORK SHEET FOR COGNITIVE RESTRUCTURING

$$A + iB \rightarrow C$$

$$A + rB \rightarrow \begin{cases} aE \text{ (Affective)} \\ bE \text{ (Behavioral)} \\ cE \text{ (Cognitive)} \end{cases}$$

Activating Event: _____

Irrational Beliefs (automatic thoughts):	Disputes (questions):	Rational Beliefs (replies):
1. _____	1. _____	1. _____
2. _____	2. _____	2. _____
3. _____	3. _____	3. _____
4. _____	4. _____	4. _____
5. _____	5. _____	5. _____

Consequences (emotions, physical discomfort):_____

_____

Effects (affective, behavioral, cognitive):_____

_____

ADVANCED HOMEWORK SHEET FOR COGNITIVE RESTRUCTURING

Activating Event _____

Irrational beliefs (automatic thoughts):

rating

1. ( ) _____

                                     rerating

_____. ( )

2. ( ) _____

_____. ( )

3. ( ) _____

_____. ( )

4. ( ) _____

_____. ( )

Rational beliefs (replies):

1. _____

                                     rating

_____. ( )

2. _____

_____. ( )

3. _____

_____. ( )

4. _____

_____

List consequences (negative emotions, physical discomfort):

    rating   rerating

1. ( ) _____( )

2. ( ) _____( )

3. ( ) _____( )

4. ( ) _____( )

List effects (affective, behavioral, or cognitive):

1. _____

2. _____

3. _____

4. _____

Directions: When experiencing unpleasant emotions, list these under Consequences and rate them (1 = minimally present, 100 = most intense possible). Now record the situation which seemed to bring them on in the Activating Event section. Next, record the irrational beliefs that you have linked to the activating event in the appropriate section and rate your degree of belief (0 = no belief, 100 = total belief). Then record the rational beliefs and rate your degree of belief in them. Rerate the irrational beliefs. Next, list the effects resulting from generating your rational replies. Then rerate the original consequences.

APPENDIX 17

THERAPIST'S EXAMPLE

I was in my office the morning before leaving on a business trip with my desk piled high with papers awaiting my attention. I began noticing the signs of gradually rising body tension, especially in my stomach. This was accompanied by feelings of depression and inertia, making it difficult to become sufficiently energized to get anything accomplished. I caught myself saying such things to myself as: "This work load is insurmountable. Others will see me as not doing my fair share and will be furious with me. I'll be fired for neglecting my responsibilities and will never find so attractive a position. If I can't keep up with this level of responsibility, it will be apparent to everyone and I'll never be promoted to a higher level in my organization. If I do manage to get away today it will surely be by neglecting something important, which I'll only remember too late, and it will spoil my trip." When I caught myself making these kinds of statements, I hastened to challenge them with such questions as "Haven't I fallen behind in my paperwork like this before? Am I so sure that there are no better positions out there waiting for me? Does being behind temporarily mean that I can't keep up with my responsibilities and that I won't be promoted? Isn't there a way to check that I've accomplished the major tasks? Would forgetting something have to spoil my trip?"

In responding to these questions which challenged my initial depressing thoughts, I answered that I have been in very similar situations in the past and that during those times I have survived falling behind in my paperwork. Even when my being swamped has come to the attention of others, there have been no negative consequences. In considering the worst possible outcome, losing my job, I can't be sure a better job isn't waiting for me elsewhere. Falling behind at

229

work does not mean I can't keep up with responsibilities. Falling behind in paperwork is not necessarily a sign of irresponsibility and certainly not a criterion for denying promotion! In addition, I am able to run a check on major tasks to be accomplished before leaving for the weekend.

APPENDIX 18

BASIC IRRATIONAL IDEAS

1. You must—yes, *must*—have sincere love and approval almost all the time from all the people you find significant.

2. You *must* prove yourself thoroughly competent, adequate, and achieving, or you *must* at least have real competence or talent at something important.

3. You have to view life as awful, terrible, horrible, or castastrophic when things do not go the way you would like them to go.

4. People who harm you or commit misdeeds rate as generally bad, wicked, or villainous individuals and you should severely blame, damn, and punish them for their sins.

5. If something seems dangerous or fearsome, you must become terribly occupied with and upset about it and make yourself anxious about it.

6. People and things should turn out better than they do and you have to view it as awful and horrible if you do not quickly find good solutions to life's hassles.

7. Emotional misery comes from external pressures and you have little ability to control your feelings or rid yourself of depression and hostility.

8. You will find it easier to avoid facing many of life's difficulties and self-responsibilities than to undertake more rewarding forms of self-discipline.

From A. A. Ellis, *Reason and Emotion in Psychotherapy*. New York: Lyle Stuart, 1962, Reprinted by permission.

9. Your past remains all-important and because something once strongly influenced your life, it has to keep determining your feelings and behavior today.

10. You can achieve happiness by inertia and inaction or by passively and uncommittedly "enjoying yourself."

11. You have to view things as awful, terrible, horrible, and castastrophic when you get seriously frustrated, treated unfairly, or rejected.

12. You must have a high degree of order or certainty to feel comfortable, or you need some supernatural power on which to rely.

13. You can give yourself a global rating as a human, and your general worth and self-acceptance depend upon the goodness of your performances and the degree to which people approve of you.

HOMEWORK SHEET FOR COGNITIVE RESTRUCTURING

$$A + iB \rightarrow C$$

$$A + rB \rightarrow \begin{cases} aE \text{ (Affective)} \\ bE \text{ (Behavioral)} \\ cE \text{ (Cognitive)} \end{cases}$$

Activating Event: Called into boss's office. Boss says, ''I have a problem with the work you turned in yesterday. Please see me in five minutes.''

Irrational beliefs (automatic thoughts):	Disputes (questions)	Rational beliefs(replies):
1. No one appreciates me.	1. Is there truly no one who appreciates me?	1. I can name several people who appreciate me.
2. Everyone will find out and think less of me.	2. Who is "everyone"? How likely is it that this will be reported to everyone? If people do find out, will	2. Our grapevine is not that efficient. I don't know for certain that finding out will make someone think less of

	they think less of me? What if they do?	me. People who matter won't.
3. I'll never get ahead.	3. Does having to do this work mean that I'll never get ahead? Do I know for certain that I'll never advance?	3. Redoing one item of work doesn't designate me for stagnation.
4. I'm incompetent.	4. Do I always do incompetent work? Does having to redo work mean I'm incompetent?	4. On occasion I've been complimented on the quality of my work. No one does their work perfectly all the time.
5. I'm going to be fired and will never find another job that will suit me.	5. What evidence is there that I will be fired for this? Do I know for certain that I couldn't find another job that would suit me?	5. No one has been fired here for such a trivial matter. There are many attractive jobs for which I could qualify. I don't have a crystal ball.

Consequences (emotions, physical discomfort):
I feel anxious. I have stomach pains. I feel frozen in my chair.
Effects (affective, behavioral, cognitive):
1. I feel less anxious. 2. My stomach pains have vanished. 3. I feel good about myself and I have regained confidence in my work. 4. I am able to get up and walk calmly to the boss's office.

CBT HOMEWORK SHEET: EXAMPLE ORIGINALLY PREPARED FOR NONDISCLOSURE TO GROUP

A. Activating Event

We're on vacation, staying with my mother-in-law. I'm already in bed and feeling sleepy. Have left B. watching the kids and drinking beer. B. comes to bed full of beer and feels like making love. I feel resistant but not entirely negative. We make love for a while; physically everything is fine, he's a good lover (by my book), but my mind is elsewhere thinking "I don't really like you/me kinds of thoughts: this is nice, but not exciting like it once was; please finish now; I'm satisfied and I have to get up in the morning to be with D. while you sleep late; why am I being so unresponsive, noninventive? I feel generally stuck in a rut; lovemaking is good; why do I never initiate it? Am I going to grow, change any more?"

iB. Irrational Beliefs

1. When lovemaking with spouse isn't exciting, it will never be again and that's cause for depression.

2. I'm the only one who gets up with D, B. never does.

3. B. shouldn't enjoy lovemaking because I'm not *really* enjoying it.

4. I should be a continually growing self-actualizing person and this should be evident through vivacity and sexual desire. If I am stuck now, it follows that I must be very anxious about this feeling.

5. I never initiate lovemaking. To initiate lovemaking is the most important way to show love for a partner.

6. I am unlikely to experience growth and change, since the feelings I have now are not new to me. This stuck feeling will always be a part of me.

C. Consequence

I feel very blue the following day. Have long talk with B., but do not feel hopeful about any self-initiated change, as I didn't know what to do.

D. Disputes

1. A lull now doesn't mean forever, does it?

2. Although I rarely request, hasn't B. gotten up with D. when asked before?

3. Are you sure of this? Is it awful and terrible that you're not really turned on? Is that a reason for B. not to enjoy himself?

4. What evidence do you have that change is not possible? Haven't you grown a lot during the past ten years of marriage? Haven't you also felt low for periods during the past ten years and then gotten out of that to something better?

5. Is sex the ultimate indicator? Don't you show love in other ways? If you're concerned about this, okay, but need it be paramount?

6. Are your present low feelings exactly the same as before? Do you expect alternating times of hibernation and growth?

rB. Rational Beliefs

1. Nothing is perfect all the time (e.g., When things don't go well for "too long," try to figure out a way to change, don't mull over failures).

2. B. will be more helpful if you ask him specifically (e.g., You must ask, let him know what you want). It's not terrible that you don't get the "perfect" amount of sleep tonight.

3. It is frustrating not to enjoy yourself as much as your partner does. I can begin to make plans to make lovemaking more desirable, exciting.

4. Again, this is an unfortunate feeling. I can make plans to begin to move out of my present hiatus and start growing again.

5. I would like to be perfect at lovemaking, but I don't need to be. B. is a loving and reasonable person and doesn't need for me to be perfect either.

6. I can still grow even though this present feeling is frustrating. I can begin to make plans for making my life more desirable.

E. Effects
(Affective)
No longer feeling blue.
(Behavioral)
Reading more on CBT (Cognitive Behavior Therapy) and more willing to use the technique again.
(Cognitive)
Just because certain situations with my husband aren't ideal doesn't
mean that I must begin to catastrophize about my marriage and my life.

APPENDIX 21

CBT HOMEWORK SHEET: EXAMPLE DONE AT HOME THAT PROMPTED SELF-DISCLOSURE IN THE GROUP

A. Activating Event:
   Disclosing something personal about my relationship with B.

iB. Irrational Beliefs:

   1. Group members and leaders will think B.'s a crazy alcoholic ogre.

   2. By association I am weak, stupid to be with him.

   3. I must have approval, respect of group members and leaders.

   4. I must have an excellent marriage relationship with B.

C. Consequence:
   Preoccupied with assignment while trying to sleep, make love, or be with D. Snapped at D. prior to writing out this sheet.

D. Disputes:

   1. Do I have any evidence that group members and leaders will sit in judgment of myself or my marriage?

   2. Do one spouse's problems equal stupidity of other spouse?

3. Is their approval more important than working these things out? What real difference will their approval or lack thereof make in my life?

4. Does "want" equal "must"?

rB. Rational Beliefs:

1. Group members and leaders will probably not be harshly judgmental.

2. As I don't see X as a weak unit even though I don't like Y, it'll probably be same here. (X and Y = another couple)

3. Though I want the approval of others, not having it is not catastrophic.

4. Again, I want a "perfect" relationship. Perfection may or may not be something to strive for, but not achieving it is not cause for despair.

E. Effects:
(affective)

1. Feeling calmer.

2. No longer irritable with D.

3. Mood improved—lighter.
(behavioral)

1. I began to write out the activating event and iBs.

2. I was able to disclose my initial homework example to the group (see Appendix H).
(cognitive)

1. I want to learn to extinguish my approval-seeking anxieties and emphasize my own ability to know what is important, ethical, and so on.

APPENDIX 22

COMPONENTS OF ASSERTIVE BEHAVIOR

1. EYE CONTACT

2. FACIAL EXPRESSION

3. GESTURES AND BODY POSTURE

4. VOICE TONE, INFLECTION, AND VOLUME

5. CONTENT

6. TIMING

APPENDIX 23

SCRIPTED ASSERTIVE SCENES

1. Situation:

You are the driver of a car that has just been flagged down by a policeman for speeding. You are attempting to explain your behavior and avoid receiving a ticket.

OFFENDER: Oh, I'm terribly sorry, officer, for going over the speed limit. I was in a great hurry.

OFFICER: Hurry? What was your rush?

OFFENDER: Actually, there's no good reason to exceed the limit and I'm sorry to have done it. I would have gotten to my destination much faster had I observed the speed limit.

OFFICER: You people have no respect for rules, they're for your own good, you know.

OFFENDER: Perfectly right, sir. These rules are for everyone's protection and I thank you for calling my attention to this. I think I've learned my lesson.

2. Situation:

You are alone at a party and have just caught the eye of someone you find attractive. You'd like to meet him/her and walk over to the person.

ENTRANCED: Hi. My name is _____. I couldn't help but notice how attractive that (article of clothing or jewelry) is that you're wearing. (Pause for response.)

ENTRANCER: I was given it as a gift by my mother.

ENTRANCED: Gee, that was thoughtful. Are you a friend of John's (name of host)?

243

I haven't known him very long but really appreciate his throwing a party. How is it that you know John?

ENTRANCER: We went to school together years ago and happened to bump into each other only by chance early this week.

ENTRANCED: Oh, that must have been a pleasant surprise. What school was it that you both attended?

APPENDIX 24

VIGNETTES FOR ASSERTIVENESS TRAINING

VIGNETTE 1

Situation
You see your physician for a persistent cough. He examines you and prescribes a medication. You ask your diagnosis, how the medication is supposed to act, and what your diagnosis is. The physician says, "You don't need to worry about that. Just take these pills and you'll feel much better."

Goal
To persevere and attempt to obtain the information you requested.

VIGNETTE 2

Situation
You are already feeling overworked when your boss gives you an extra assignment that you feel could be given to someone else just as easily.

Goal
To attempt to turn down your boss's assignment while explaining your reasons.

VIGNETTE 3

Situation
Friends of yours invite you to go on a picnic but end up asking you to do most of the shopping and cooking. You accept, expecting it to be a joint venture (you don't have the time or the inclination to do all the work). You decide to speak to them in advance of the picnic date.

Goal
To preserve the friendship but want to back out of the chores you have already agreed to do.

VIGNETTE 4

Situation
A person working under you has not been doing satisfactory work. You decide to speak privately with the person.

Goal
To be clear about your dissatisfaction with your subordinate's performance yet not be punishing or blaming.

VIGNETTE 5

Situation
A friend of yours is perpetually late. He/she has just arrived late again, for dinner this time. The meal you've prepared is slightly dried out as a result, having been kept warm in the oven.

Goal
To express your dissatisfaction for this and past incidents while still allowing for an explanation from your friend.

VIGNETTE 6

Situation
Someone with a romantic interest in you asks you out and you don't want to go.

Goal
To turn him/her down gently but not leave yourself open for further invitations because you're not at all interested in him/her romantically.

VIGNETTE 7

Situation
You meet an interesting new person and want to get to know him/her better.

Goal

To take the initiative to arrange another meeting.

VIGNETTE 8

Situation

Your spouse, family member, or roommate is not doing his/her share of the work around the house. You are feeling "unfaired against."

Goal

To specify what you are unhappy about and what changes you're requesting in a firm but not unfriendly manner.

VIGNETTE 9

Situation

You have been seeing someone steadily for several months and have a close and intimate relationship. Recently you have noticed that your friend is acting somewhat cool and is not seeking your company as frequently. You decide to speak with him/her.

Goal

To share your perception and to maximize your chances of getting an honest answer.

VIGNETTE 10

Situation

You are at a party. You have decided that you would prefer not to drink or eat for personal reasons, but the host is pressuring you to eat or imbibe.

Goal

To turn down your host's offerings firmly but politely.

VIGNETTE 11

Situation

You are in the middle of a job interview. You are really interested in the job, but the salary they're offering is lower than you are willing to accept.

Goal

To get them to increase the salary offer.

VIGNETTE 12

Situation

You have just spent the evening out for dinner with a person you've only just met. The person wants to continue the evening in your or his/her apartment. You wish to end the evening now. The other person is persistent.

Goal

You'd like to see him/her again and do not rule out a romantic relationship in the future, but you are firm that tonight is not "the night."

VIGNETTE 13

Situation

You've heard that a colleague has been bad-mouthing your work. You want to speak to him/her.

Goal

You want to stop this behavior without creating additional bad feelings or making a "scene."

VIGNETTE 14

Situation

An old friend has just come in from out of town and wants to meet you for lunch. You have an important business engagement. The friend begins inspiring guilt.

Goal

You do not want to "cave in" and cancel your business appointment but you do want to preserve your friendship.

VIGNETTE 15

Situation

You've inadvertently missed a luncheon appointment with a dear friend. The friend expresses much hurt and believes that you've lost interest in him/her.

Goal

You want to reassure your friend of the good feelings you have for him/her.

VIGNETTE 16

Situation

A couple that you don't know very well is visiting your town and calling to ask if they can stay with you for the weekend. You have many plans, several of which will be significantly hampered by house guests.

Goal

Without being rude, you want to talk them out of staying at your house.

APPENDIX 25

ASSERTIVE BEHAVIOR LOG

Please recount below a situation in which you behaved assertively or in which you wish you had behaved assertively.

  1. Briefly describe the situation below and your feelings.

            Please list your anxiety level on a scale of 0–100* _____

  2. What did you say and/or do? _____
_____

                                            Anxiety level _____

  3. How did you feel afterward? _____
_____

                                            Anxiety level _____

  4. If given another opportunity, would you have said or done anything differently?
     Yes ( ) No ( )
     If yes, specify. _____
_____

  5. How do you think your words and/or behavior were interpreted by the other person? _____
_____

*0 = no anxiety; 100 = incapacitating anxiety.

PROBLEM-SOLVING HOMEWORK SHEET

1. Problem Identification
   a. Background (specify): _____
   _____
   b. Detail problem situation: _____
   _____

2. Goal formation (How will you know when you've solved the problem?):
   _____
   _____

3. Generation of alternatives (Brainstorm as many alternatives as you can without censoring them):
   a. _____
   b. _____
   c. _____
   d. _____
   e. _____

4. Evaluate alternatives in terms of their probable consequences:

	Pros	Cons	Rate potential effectiveness (1 = least; 5 = most)
a.	_____	_____	_____
b.	_____	_____	_____
c.	_____	_____	_____
d.	_____	_____	_____
e.	_____	_____	_____

5. Decision making. Based on evaluation rating (step 4), choose the most likely alternative(s):

_____

6. Verification for appropriateness of selected alternative. Is this alternative likely to reach your goal? If not, return to step 3. Yes ( ) No ( )

_____

7. Preparation for implementation. What steps are necessary to implement the chosen alternative?

_____

8. Implementation. Specify outcome in terms of the identified problem.

_____

APPENDIX 27

COMPLETED PROBLEM-SOLVING HOMEWORK SHEET

1. Problem identification

   a. Background (specify): Charles and I dated for four years. It ended last week.

   b. Detail problem situation: I'm shy, hate the dating scene, and only stayed with Charles so long to avoid having to return to dating.

2. Goal formation (How will you know when you've solved the problem?):
   I want to increase my opportunities to meet eligible men.

3. Generation of alternatives (Brainstorm as many alternatives as you can without censoring them):

   a. Take a university course.

   b. Join the "Y."

   c. Go to church "singles" functions.

   d. Join a ski club in winter, beach house in summer.

   e. Ask friends to help in meeting men.

   f. Ask Charles for help in meeting men.

   g. Ask an eligible male friend from work out for a drink.

4. Evaluate alternatives in terms of their probable consequences:
Rate potential effectiveness (1 = least/5 = most)

	Pros	Cons	
a.	Could meet someone ambitious	Dislike night courses, exhausting	2
b.	Like athletics	Most activities not coed	1
c.	Like religion, know of such a group	Feel shy in new settings	4
d.	Many singles at these activities	Too competitive	2
e.	Easily done	I doubt it yields anything.	3
f.	Charles has many friends.	He wouldn't help and they're mostly duds.	1
g.	I'd love to go out with Joe.	I lack the nerve.	3

5. Decision making. Based on evaluation rating (item d), choose the most likely alternative(s):

Alternative C

6. Verification for appropriateness of selected alternative. Is this alternative likely to reach your goal? If not, return to step 3. Yes ( ) No ( )

7. Preparation for implementation. What steps are necessary to implement the chosen alternative?

(1) Call for information

(2) Keep free time

(3) Get appropriate clothes

(4) Notify my pastor of my plans

8. Implementation. Specify outcome in terms of the identified problem:

I met more friends and their friends. I've also been invited to nonchurch functions. This increased my chances of meeting eligible men.

APPENDIX 28

EXAMPLE OF COMPLETED GOAL SHEET
FOR FINAL INTERVIEW

1. Goals Met

  A. Problem 1: When Bill is out of town, I'm in constant fear that my daughter
and I will have another terrible fight.

  Goal 1: To worry less about my temper when her father is away from
home

  Skills utilized in meeting goal 1:

    1. Assertion with Janet.

    2. Cognitive restructuring (anticatastrophizing).

    3. Problem solving about how to get her father involved in disciplining
her.

  B. Problem 2: Persistent sleep problems.

  Goal 2: To fall asleep quicker and not wake up as often

  Skills utilized in meeting goal 2:

    1. Cognitive restructuring about my worries, even the worry about being
sleepless

    2. Relaxation exercises before sleep (DMR & BRR)

2. Goals Requiring Additional Work

A. Problem 1: Unhappiness whenever I'm at work or even when thinking about work

Goal 1: To feel less bad about work

Skills appropriate for meeting goal 1:

1. To be more assertive with my boss

2. Problem solving how to get a promotion

3. Cognitive restructuring for my feelings about being taken advantage of and being a scapegoat

B. Problem 2: My boyfriend is treating me more like a friend.

Goal 2: Get my boyfriend to be more affectionate

Skills appropriate for meeting goal 2:

1. To assert myself with Bob at a suitable place and time

2. To problem solve for other ways

3. To use cognitive restructuring so that I won't care so much

4. To use relaxation techniques instead of eating when I'm insecure about Bob (He's more affectionate when I'm thinner!)

WORKSHEET FOR REMAINING PROBLEMS

Goals Requiring Additional Work

A. Problem 1: _____

Goal 1: _____

Skills appropriate for meeting goal 1:

1. _____

2. _____

3. _____

B. Problem 2: _____

Goal 2: _____

Skills appropriate for meeting goal 2:

1. _____

2. _____

3. _____

INDIVIDUAL GOAL SHEET FOR FINAL INTERVIEW

I. Goals Met

  A. Goal 1: _____

  _____

    Skills utilized in meeting goal 1:

      1. _____

      2. _____

      3. _____

  B. Goal 2: _____

  _____

    Skills utilized in meeting goal 2:

      1. _____

      2. _____

      3. _____

  C. Goal 3: _____

  _____

    Skills utilized in meeting goal 3:

      1. _____

      2. _____

      3. _____

II. Goals Requiring Additional Work

  A. Goal 1: _____

  _____

    Skills appropriate for meeting goal 1:

      1. _____

    2. _____

    3. _____

B. Goal 2: _____

_____

Skills appropriate for meeting goal 2:

    1. _____

    2. _____

    3. _____

C. Goal 3: _____

_____

Skills appropriate for meeting goal 3:

    1. _____

    2. _____

    3. _____

APPENDIX 31

LOG OF PROBLEM SITUATIONS AND SKILLS EMPLOYED

Situation 1	Negative emotions	SUD* levels (Before)	Skills used	SUD levels (After)
Situation 2	Negative emotions	SUD levels (Before)	Skills used	SUD levels (After)
Situation 3	Negative emotions	SUD levels (Before)	Skills used	SUD levels (After)

*Subjective units of discomfort; 0 = no discomfort, 100 = maximum level.

Situation 4	Negative emotions	SUD levels (Before)	Skills used	SUD levels (After)
Situation 5	Negative emotions	SUD levels (Before)	Skills used	SUD levels (After)

INDEX

ABCDE Paradigm for Cognitive
    Restructuring, 78
    introduction to, 82–87
Active listening, 133–134, 136–137
Aggression, 117–118
Altruism, 33–34
Anxiety, 1, 9, 17, 21
    assertion and, 118–119
    cognitive restructuring module, 68
    competency/mastery scenes, 79–80
    relaxation and, 41–42, 52
    screening procedure and, 27
    test anxiety, 22–23
A/P sheets. *See* Attendance/Performance
    Record and Contract
Assertion techniques, 126–129
Assertion-training module
    bibliotherapy for, 6
    coping skills program and, 4
Assertion-training module (Session 8),
    113–123
    administrative tasks in, 114–115
    aggression/assertion definition,
        117–118
    assertion role, 118–119
    bibliotherapy, 116

Assertion-training module (Session 8)
    (*cont.*)
    cognitive restructuring and, 119–120
    discussion in, 120–121
    feedback, 121–122
    homework, 122
    homework question and answer, 115
    introduction to, 113–114
    overview of, 113
    Personal Reminder Form, 122
    role playing in, 121–122
    whole-body relaxation, 115–116
Assertion-training module (Session 9),
    125–132
    administrative tasks in, 126
    assertion techniques explained, 126–
        129
    feedback, 130–131, 132
    homework, 131–132
    homework question and answer, 126
    introduction to, 125–126
    overview of, 125
    Personal Reminder Form, 132
    repetition, 127–128
    role playing in, 129–130, 131
    videotaping, 130, 131

Assertion–training module (Session 10), 133–140
  active listening, 136–137
  administrative tasks in, 134
  bibliotherapy, 134–135
  feedback, 139
  goals, 139
  homework, 139, 140
  homework question and answer, 134
  "I" messages, 135–136
  introduction to, 133–134
  overview of, 133
  Personal Reminder Form, 140
  role playing, 137–139
Assertion–training module (Session 11), 141–147
  administrative tasks in, 142
  bibliotherapy, 142–143
  cognitive restructuring techniques in, 143–144
  conflict resolution, 144–145
  feedback, 146
  homework, 146–147
  homework question and answer, 142
  introduction to, 141–142
  overview of, 141
  Personal Reminder Form, 146
  role playing, 145
Assertive Behavior Log (ABL), 122
Assertiveness training, 19
Assessment tools, 31
Attendance, 36
Attendance/Performance Record and Contract
  explanation of, 39–40
  relaxation module, 42–43, 45, 49, 50–52
  screening interview, 35–36
Automatic thoughts, 70–71, 78
  assertion–training module and, 143–144
  categorization of, 81–82
  externalization-of-voices technique and, 71–73, 102–103
  generation of, 73–75
  group work on, 94–95
Aversive imagery therapy, 16

Behavior therapy, 13
  coping skills training and, 11, 14–15
  groups and, 19
  shift in, 15–18
Belief systems, 83–87
Benson's relaxation response, 42, 45–46
Bibliotherapy
  assertion–training module, 116, 120–121, 134–135, 142–143
  coping skills program, 6–7
Booster sessions, 177–179
  closing session and, 176
  homework assignment, 179
  introduction to, 177–179
  overview of, 177
  preparation for, 170
  problems remaining, 178–179
  progress/accomplishments, 178
  reorientation, 178
Broken record technique, 127–128
Buddy system
  homework assignments and, 46–47
  relaxation module, 50
  screening interview, 37
Burns books, 50

Closing session, preview of, 161–163
Closing session (Session 14), 165–170
  administrative tasks in, 167
  booster session preparation in, 170
  exit interview preparation in, 169
  feedback in, 168–169
  fees, 167
  homework, 170
  homework question and answer, 167
  introduction to, 165–166
  overview of, 165
  problem review in, 168
  success experiences, 167–168
Closing session (Session 15), 171–176
  booster session and, 176
  feedback in, 174–176
  goal development and planning in, 174
  goal strategy formulation in, 173–174
  introduction to, 171–172
  orientation, 172
  overview of, 171
  review in, 172–173

Coaching, 15
Cognitive behavior therapy (CBT), 13, 64
    advantages of, vii
    coping skills program and, 9–23
    group therapy, viii, 19, 88
    research in, 7
    theory and, 68–69
Cognitive behavior therapy homework
    sheet, 94–96
Cognitive distortion
    automatic thoughts and, 81–82
    nonassertive behavior and, 143
Cognitive restructuring, 13
    assertion training and, 119–120, 143–
        144
    bibliotherapy for, 6
    coping skills program, 4
    effectiveness and, 21
    group format, 19
Cognitive restructuring module, 63–76
    administrative tasks, 65
    automatic thoughts, 70–71, 73–75
    externalization-of-voices technique,
        71–73
    feedback, 75
    homework, 75, 76
    homework question and answer, 65–
        66
    introduction to, 64
    overview of, 63
    pairing scenes with DMR, 66–68
    Personal Reminder Form, 76
    teaching skills of, 70
    theory and, 68–69
Cognitive skills enhancement (Session
    4), 77–89
    ABCDE paradigm, 82–87
    administrative tasks in, 78
    automatic thoughts categorization, 81–
        82
    feedback in, 89
    group practice of, 87–88
    homework, 89
    homework question and answer, 78–
        80
    introduction to, 77–78
    overview of, 77
    Personal Reminder Form, 89
    tensing elimination, 80–81

Cognitive skills enhancement (Session
    5), 91–97
    administrative tasks in, 92
    CBT homework sheet, 94–96
    differential relaxation, 94
    feedback, 96
    homework, 96, 97
    homework question and answer, 92–
        93
    introduction to, 92
    overview of, 91
    Personal Reminder Form, 97
Cognitive skills enhancement (Session
    6), 99–105
    administrative tasks in, 100
    externalization-of-voices technique in,
        102–104
    feedback, 104
    homework, 104–105
    homework question and answer, 100–
        101
    introduction to, 99–100
    overview of, 99
    relaxation material, 101
Cognitive therapy, 13
    copying skills and, 11, 12–13
    groups and, 19
Commitment, 34
Confidentiality, 38
Conflict resolution, 144–145. See also
        Problem-solving approach
Content, 120
Coping model, 10
Coping role models, 33
Coping skills program
    bibliotherapy, 6–7
    case illustration of, 4–6
    cognitive behavior therapy and, 9–23
    coping model in, 10
    development of, 1
    effectiveness rationale, 20–23
    group therapy in, 19–20
    modules in, 3–4
    origin of, 11–18
    practitioner in, 1
    psychoeducational model, 10–11
    research in, 7–8
    screening procedure, 25–40
    sequence of, 6

Coping skills program (*cont.*)
  setting of, 2–3
  variety of techniques in, 18
Covert sensitization, 16

Decision making, 152
Deep muscle relaxation (DMR), 52–54
  pairing scenes with, 66–68
  tensing elimination, 80–81
Dependence, 33
Deposits, 37–38
Depression, 1, 9, 21
  assertion and, 118–119
  cognitive restructuring module, 68
  learned helplessness concept and, 21–22
Desensitization, 16
  group format and, 19
Differential relaxation, 94
Disarming. *See* Fogging
Distortions. *See* Cognitive distortions
DMR. *See* Deep muscle relaxation (DMR)

Education, 10–11
Evaluation. *See* Success
Evaluation (formal), 30–31
Exit interview, 169
Expectations, 26
Externalization-of-voices technique, 71–73, 102–104
Eye contact, 119–120

Facial expression, 120
Fear-of-being-a-casualty myth, 35
Feedback
  assertion–training modules, 121–122, 130–131, 132, 139, 146
  closing sessions, 168–169, 174–176
  cognitive restructuring and, 75
  cognitive skills enhancement, 89, 96, 104
  midway evaluation, 110, 111
  problem-solving modules, 155, 163
  relaxation modules, 47, 61
Fees
  closing sessions, 167
  screening interview, 37–38
Final interview, 172
Fogging, 128–129, 138
Follow-up sessions, 177–179

Formal evaluation, 30–31
Freud, S., 11, 12

Genetic factors, 11
George Washington University Health Plan, 1
Goals
  assertion–training modules, 120–121, 139, 145
  closing session, 172–174
  midway evaluation, 109–110
  problem-solving module, 152, 155
  relaxation module, 44–45
  role playing and, 131
  screening procedure, 26, 32
Ground rules, 35–39
Groups, viii
  coping skills program and, 19–20
  individual therapy versus, 33–34, 35
  problem-solving module, 159–161
  screening procedure and, 26
  setting for, 2–3
  size of, 2

Homework
  assertion–training modules, 115, 122, 126, 131–132, 134, 139, 140, 142, 146–147
  attendance interview, 36–37
  booster session, 179
  closing session, 167, 170
  cognitive restructuring module, 65–66, 75, 76
  cognitive skills enhancement, 79–80, 89, 92–93, 96, 97, 100–101, 104–105
  problem-solving module, 151, 155–156, 158, 163, 164
  relaxation modules, 46–47, 48, 50, 60–61
Hypnosis, 16

Identification, 34
"I" messages, 133–134, 135–136, 138
Independence, 33
Individual therapy and sessions
  group therapy versus, 33–34, 35
  midway evaluation, 107–111. *See also* Midway evaluation
  screening procedure, 28

Instigation therapy, 15–16
Instinct theory, 11
Insurance, 18
Intelligence, 28
Interdependence, 33
Irrational, definitions, 87
Irrational beliefs, ABCDE paradigm, 83–87

Learned helplessness, 21–22
Least-expensive, least-effective myth, 35
Length of session, 2

Mastery model
   coping model compared, 10
   effectiveness of, 20
Medical model, 12, 18
   psychoeducational model and, 11
Medication, 28
Meditation, 45–46
Message content, 120
Midway evaluation, 107–111
   administrative tasks in, 108
   discussion in, 108–109
   feedback in, 110, 111
   homework, 110–111
   homework question and answer, 108
   introduction to, 107, 108
   overview of, 107
   Personal Reminder Form, 111
   review of goals in, 109–110
Motivation, 28

Name game, 43

One-way mirrors, 3
Orientation
   problem-solving appraoch, 152–153
   relaxation module, 42–43
   success rates and, 26

Participation, 38–39
Patient selection, 29–30
Peer learning, 33
Penalties, 37, 39
Personal Reminder Form
   assertion–training modules, 122, 132, 140, 146
   cognitive restructuring module, 76
   cognitive skills enhancement, 89, 97, 104

Personal Reminder Form (cont.)
   midway evaluation, 111
   problem-solving module, 155, 163
   relaxation module, 47–48, 50, 61
Phobias, 17, 22
Posture, 120
Practitioner, 1
Pregroup interview. See Screening procedure
Pretreatment Questionnaire, 27, 30
Prevention, 16
Problem behaviors, 37, 39
Problem-solving approach
   coping skills program, 4
   See also Conflict resolution
Problem-solving module (Session 12), 149–156
   administrative tasks in, 150–151
   explanation of process in, 151–153
   feedback, 155
   goals in, 155
   homework, 155–156
   homework question and answer, 151
   introduction to, 149–150, 151
   overview of, 149
   Personal Reminder Form, 155
   role playing, 153–155
Problem-solving module (Session 13), 157–164
   administrative tasks in, 158
   feedback, 163
   group exercise for, 159–161
   homework, 163, 164
   homework question and answer, 158
   introduction to, 157–158
   overview of, 157
   Personal Reminder Form, 163
   preview of closing sessions, 161–163
   problem identification in, 158–159
Progressive Muscle Relaxation, 52
Promptness, 36
Psychoeducational approach, 10–11
   behavior therapy and, 14–15
   resistance to, 17–18
Psychopathology, 14
Psychosis, 28
Psychotherapy
   coping model and, 10
   psychoeducational model and, 11
Public commitment, 34

Rational, definitions, 86
Rational behavior training, 13
Rational beliefs, 83–87
Rational-emotive therapy (RET), 13, 64
  advantages of, vii
  coping skills and, 12–13
  group therapy, viii
Rational psychotherapy, 13
Rational restructuring, 13
Referrals
  formal evaluation, 30
  group treatment, 26
  patient selection, 29
  screening procedure, 25
Relaxation
  cognitive skills enhancement, 101
  coping skills and, 20
  differential relaxation, 94
  group format and, 19
  midway evaluation, 108–109
  problems in, 93, 100–101
  tensing elimination, 80–81
  whole-body relaxation, 115–116
Relaxation module (Session 1), 41–48
  A/P sheet, 45
  Benson's Relaxation Response, 45–46
  coping skills program, 3–4
  feedback in, 47
  first warm-up exercise, 43
  goals, 44–45
  homework, 46–47, 48
  introduction to, 41–42
  orientation, 42–43
  overview of, 41
  Personal Reminder Form 47–48
  second warm-up exercise, 43–44
Relaxation module (Session 2), 49–61
  A/P sheets, 49, 50–52
  deep muscle relaxation, 52–54
  feedback, 61
  homework, 50, 60–61
  introduction to, 49–50
  overview of, 49
  Personal Reminder Form, 61
  script for, 54–60
  Subjective Units of Discomfort (SUD)
    concept, 52, 53
Relaxation Practice Log, 50–51
Reorientation, 178

Repetition, 127–128
Research
  coping skills program, 7–8
  screening procedure, 25
Rogers, Carl, 12
Role models, 33
Role playing
  assertion-training modules, 114, 121–
    122, 129–130, 131, 137–139, 144,
    145
  problem-solving module, 153–155
Role playing/reverse role playing,
    71–73

Screening interview, 31–40
  assessment tools in, 31
  Attendance/Performance Record and
    Contract, 39–40
  clarifications in, 34–35
  description of group, 32–33
  discussion in, 31–32
  goals development, 32
  ground rule explanation in, 35–39
  group versus individual treatment,
    33–34
  patient preparation for, 31
Screening procedure, 25–40
  formal evaluation, 30–31
  introduction to, 25–29
  overview of, 25
  patient selection, 29–30
  rationale for, 28–29
  screening interview, 31–40. See also
    Screening interview
Secrets game, 43–44
Self-disclosure, 44
Self-efficacy, 21–22
Semantic therapy, 13
Six-month follow-up session, 177–179
Solitary-use myth, 35
Subjective Units of Discomfort (SUD)
  concept, 52, 53
Success
  booster session, 178
  closing sessions, 167–168, 172–173
  orientation and, 26
SUD. See Subjective Units of Discomfort
    (SUD)
Systematic rational restructuring, 13

Test anxiety, 22–23
Testing, 31
Theory, 68–69
Third-party payers, 18
Thought disorders, 28
Timing, 120
Touchy-feely myth, 34–35

Transcendental meditation, 45
Twelve-month follow-up session, 179

Vicarious learning, 33
Videotaping, 130, 131, 138
Voice tone, 120

Whole-body relaxation, 115–116